COMPANION TO
CLINICAL ANAESTHESIA EXAMS

C. F. Corke MBBS, MRCP(UK), FANZCA, FFICANZCA

I. J. B. Jackson MBChB, FRCA

SECOND EDITION

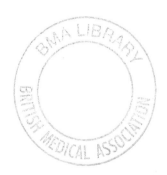

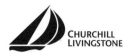
CHURCHILL
LIVINGSTONE

EDINBURGH LONDON NEW YORK PHILADELPHIA ST LOUIS SYDNEY TORONTO 2002

CHURCHILL LIVINGSTONE
An imprint of Harcourt Publishers Limited

© Harcourt Publishers Limited 2002

 is a registered trademark of Harcourt Publishers Limited

The right of Charles F. Corke and Ian J.B. Jackson to be identified as authors of this work has been asserted by them in accordance with the Copyright, Designs and Patents Act 1988

First published 1994
Second edition 2002

ISBN 0 443 07104 7

British Library Cataloguing in Publication Data
A catalogue record for this book is available from the British Library

Library of Congress Cataloging in Publication Data
A catalog record for this book is available from the Library of Congress

Note
Medical knowledge is constantly changing. As new information becomes available, changes in treatment, procedures, equipment and the use of drugs become necessary. The authors and the publishers have, as far as it is possible, taken care to ensure that the information given in this text is accurate and up to date. However, readers are strongly advised to confirm that the information, especially with regard to drug usage, complies with the latest legislation and standards of practice.

The
Publisher's
Policy is to use
**paper manufactured
from sustainable forests**

Printed in China by the RDC Group

Preface

FIRST EDITION

Extensive reading of the leading anaesthetic texts is essential for success in clinical anaesthetic examinations but these texts usually cover topics in such detail that memorization and subsequent recall of important points can be difficult.

In this book the Answer Plans, which are presented in note or essay plan form, aim to help candidates to identify clearly important points of various anaesthetic topics. This system should be extended by the candidate to other subjects as they revise them. It is essential for a full and clear examination answer (in both written and oral examinations) that all the important points are covered in a logical order, and the ability to reproduce a good plan is fundamental to this.

In addition, candidates should consider whether they can competently discuss the points included in the Answer Plan lists and should revise further any areas of weakness from leading texts.

The Practical Clinical Section includes systematic approaches to the interpretation of ECGs, chest X-rays, lung function tests and blood gas results. Features of and criteria for some of the more common abnormalities are described.

Specimen viva questions on clinical anaesthesia are included in the Viva Questions section. It is intended that candidates should use these questions to practise oral examination technique with a colleague to improve their presentation. This section should also highlight areas of weakness that the candidate should revise.

Finally there is a bibliography of useful and important references to anaesthetic literature which the well-prepared candidate would be well advised to have read.

While this book is particularly aimed at those candidates preparing for the new Part III FRCA examination it will also be of value to those taking the Part I FRCA examination.

Geelong and York   C.F.C
1994   I.J.B.J

SECOND EDITION

In this second edition, the concise approach of the first edition has been preserved. The content has been updated to reflect the significant changes that have occurred in anaesthesia over the last five years.

An entirely new Glossary section has been added and is designed to assist candidates in gaining a concise understanding of a wide range of terms and principles associated with anaesthetic practice.

We have been encouraged by the many registrars who have told us that the first edition of this book helped them prepare for their examinations. We are delighted to have been able to provide this assistance and hope that this second edition will be even more useful to future candidates.

Geelong and York   C.F.C.
2001   I.J.B.J.

Abbreviations

ABE	actual base excess
ABG	arterial blood gas
ACD	acid-citrate-dextrose
ADH	antidiuretic hormone
AF	atrial fibrillation
ALA	aminolaevulinic acid
A-P	antero-posterior
ARDS	adult respiratory distress syndrome
ASD	atrioseptal defect
BMI	body mass index
BMR	basal metabolic rate
BP	blood pressure
BPt	boiling point
CAPP	coronary artery perfusion pressure
CAT	computed axial tomography
CBF	cerebral blood flow
CCF	congestive cardiac failure
CMV	cytomegalovirus
CNS	central nervous system
CO	cardiac output
COAD	chronic obstructive airways disease
COP	colloid oncotic pressure
CPAP	continuous positive airway pressure
CPD	citrate phosphate dextrose
CPP	cerebral perfusion pressure
CPK	creatinine phosphokinase
CSF	cerebrospinal fluid
CT	computed tomography
CV	closing volume
CVP	central venous pressure
CVS	cardiovascular system
CXR	chest X-ray
DI	diabetes insipidus
DNA	did not attend

2,3-DPG	2,3-diphosphoglycerate
DVT	deep venous thrombosis
EBV	Epstein–Barr virus
ECG	electrocardiogram
EEG	electroencephalogram
EMG	electromyograph
ERV	expiratory reserve volume
FEV_1	forced expiratory volume in 1 second
FFP	fresh frozen plasma
F_iO_2	inspired oxygen fraction
FRC	functional residual capacity
FVC	forced vital capacity
GABA	gamma aminobutyric acid
GFR	glomerular filtration rate
GIS	gastrointestinal system
GTN	glycerol trinitrate
HFJV	high frequency jet ventilation
HFPPV	high frequency positive pressure ventilation
HIV	human immunodeficiency virus
HR	heart rate
IC	inspiratory capacity
ICP	intracranial pressure
ICU	intensive care unit
I:E	inspiration:expiration ratio
IgE	immunoglobulin E
IMV	intermittent mandatory volume
IPPV	intermittent positive pressure ventilation
IRV	inspiratory reserve volume
IV	intravenous
IVC	inferior vena cava
LAP	left atrial pressure
LBBB	left bundle branch block
LCW	left cardiac work
LDH	lactate dehydrogenase
LMN	lower motor neurone
LOS	lower oesophageal sphincter
LVEDP	left ventricular end diastolic pressure
LVSW	left ventricular stroke work
MAC	minimum alveolar concentration
MAOI	monoamine oxidase inhibitors
MAP	mean arterial pressure
MBC	maximum breathing capacity
MRI	magnetic resonance imaging
NMDA	N-methyl-D-aspartate
NSAID	non-steroidal anti-inflammatory drug
O_2CT	oxygen content

ORL	orphan opioid receptor
P-A	postero-anterior
PAEDP	pulmonary artery end diastolic pressure
PAFC	pulmonary artery flotation catheter
PAWP	pulmonary artery wedge pressure
PBG	porphobilinogen
PCA	patient controlled analgesia
PDA	patent ductus arteriosus
PDPH	post dural pucture headache
PEEP	positive end expiratory pressure
PEFR	peak expiratory flow rate
PTC	post tetanic count
PVR	pulmonary vascular resistance
RBBB	right bundle branch block
RCW	right cardiac work
RV	residual volume
RVSW	right ventricular stroke work
RPP	rate pressure product
SAGM	saline adenine glucose mannitol
SBC	standard bicarbonate concentration
SBE	standard base excess
SGOT	serum glutamic-oxaloacetic transaminase
SIADH	syndrome of inappropriate ADH secretion
SIMV	synchronized intermittent mandatory volume
SSRI	selective serotonin reuptake inhibitors
SV	stroke volume
SVP	saturated vapour pressure
SVR	systemic vascular resistance
TBI	traumatic brain injury
TIVA	total intravenous anaesthesia
TLC	total lung capacity
TOF	train of four
UMN	upper motor neurone
UV	ultraviolet
VC	vital capacity
V_D	dead space
VIC	vaporizer in circuit
VOC	vaporizer out of circuit
VSD	ventricular septal defect
V_T	tidal volume

Contents

Answer plans

INTRODUCTION

The Answer Plans cover some of the major areas with which an examination candidate should be conversant. Invaluable as revision aids, the main emphasis of these plans is to teach a technique that helps ensure major aspects of a topic are not omitted from examination answers. They are not, and should not be considered as, a substitute for major anaesthetic texts and review articles.

The topics covered are inevitably selective but are intended to include most of the important areas of clinical anaesthesia, particularly those popular in examinations. The anatomical topics have been restricted to the major areas of interest to anaesthetists including details of regional anaesthetic techniques and the appropriate applied anatomy. Diagrams, where included, have intentionally been kept as simple as possible so that they might realistically be reproduced within the time restraints of the written or oral examination.

Candidates should attempt to structure their answers to both oral and written questions. The essay plans help with this process but it should be remembered that there are one or two classic structures that they can be superimposed on. For questions about how you would anaesthetize a particular problem case the candidate should consider the structure in Table 1.1.

It is also important to interpret the question correctly so it should be read carefully at least twice. The candidate must understand what the examiners wish to be answered before embarking on an essay or a reply in a viva. There are some key words that the candidate should look for in each question; advice on how to interpret these is given in Table 1.2.

Time is short during written examinations and candidates must plan to present clear concise answers, containing all the relevant details, within the time available. Recall and formulation of essay plans while working under stress in an examination situation is essential. Written examinations, and in particular their completion, is rather like managing an operating session – if even 5 minutes extra time is spent on each of the first five cases, the last case may need to be cancelled! The candidate cannot write for just 5 minutes

Table 1.1 Management of patient for anaesthesia – general outline

Preoperative
- Visit the patient
- Assessment with attention to general problems
  — drugs
  — allergies
  — previous anaesthetic history
  — past medical history
  — family history
  — loose teeth, presence of crowns, etc.
  — time since last ate or drank
  — potential intubation problems
  — current medical history
- Assessment with attention to problems specific to presenting complaint
- Examination of patient
- Appropriate investigations
- Premedication
- Explanation to patient of anaesthetic technique to be used/consent
- Establish weight of patient (important particularly in questions about regional anaesthesia)

Anaesthetic room
- Equipment checks
- Establish monitoring
- Establish IV access

Induction
- Drugs used
- Special techniques

Maintenance
- Monitoring
- Drugs used
- Fluids used
- Equipment used
- Special techniques

Reversal
- Technique
- Drugs used

Recovery/postoperative management
- Instructions for immediate recovery
- Postoperative analgesia
- Intravenous fluids
- Oxygen therapy
- Destination e.g. ward, HDU or ICU

on the last question and expect to pass; therefore rigorous control must be kept on the time spent on each question. Each question must be answered and candidates should beware of the trap where extra time is spent on one question because it covers a topic they understand well.

Table 1.2 Interpretation of key words

Compare	look for similarities and differences
Contrast	set in opposition in order to bring out differences
Criticize	give your judgement and back this by a discussion of the evidence; be sure to bring out negative points
Define	give the precise meaning of
Describe	give a detailed account of
Discuss	investigate by argument, debate giving reasons, the pros and cons
Explain	make plain, account for or interpret
Illustrate	make clear by examples (or may mean use a diagram to clarify)
Justify	show adequate grounds for decisions; be sure to bring out positive points
Outline	give the main features of
Relate	show how things are connected to each other and how they affect each other

ANATOMICAL AND PHYSIOLOGICAL DIFFERENCES

PAEDIATRIC

Airway

- Large head in relation to body
- Wider jaw angle than adult (140° vs 120° in adult)
- Large tongue in contact with palate = nasal breathing
- Anterior and higher larynx (C3/4 vs C5/6 in adult)
- U-shaped epiglottis
- Cricoid (subglottis) narrower than larynx
- Small radius endotracheal tubes have significant resistance

Respiratory

- $\dot{V}_{O_2}/kg$ is twice that in adult
- Predominant diaphragmatic respiration (vs intercostal)
- Functional residual capacity (FRC) < closing volume (CV), therefore closure on normal expiration (note FRC has been shown to exceed CV by 6 years of age)
- Short alveolar time constants
- Poor respiratory control with liability to apnoea (especially under anaesthesia in those aged <6/12 and particularly in premature infants)
- Small tidal volume so apparatus dead space must be minimal or alveolar ventilation will be impaired
- Rapid respiratory rate in newborn (30–40 breaths/min)

Cardiovascular system (CVS)

- Increased cardiac index; cardiac output maintained by increase in pulse rate rather than increase in stroke volume
- Increased haemoglobin (normal 18 g/100 ml in neonate)
- Increased O_2 affinity (HbF) until 3/12 (HbF constitutes 75% of haemoglobin at birth)
- Tendency to revert to fetal circulation in neonates who become hypoxic
- Tendency to bradycardia in response to hypoxia, and pronounced oculocardiac and diving reflexes
- Difficult venous access, particularly at 18–24/12
- Increased percentage body water (ml/kg) compared to adult

Temperature

- Tendency to hypothermia: high surface area, little subcutaneous fat, poor homoeostatic reflexes (thermoneutral environment 35°C in first 24 h then 32°C)
- Brown fat utilized to maintain temperature (non-shivering thermogenesis)

Metabolism

- Tendency to hypoglycaemia

Neuromuscular

- Sensitivity to non-depolarizing neuromuscular blockers and resistant to suxamethonium during first month

Central nervous system (CNS)

- Liable to central anticholinergic syndrome
- Psychological factors
- Spinal cord terminates at L3/4 (L1/2 in adult)
- Predictable spread with caudal injection (variable in adult)

MATERNAL

Respiratory

- Increased minute volume (rate and tidal volume)
- Hypocarbia ($P\text{co}_2$ 4 kPa vs 5.3 kPa in non-pregnant)
- Reduced airway resistance (? progesterone effect)
- Reduced FRC
- Reduced expiratory reserve volume
- Increased $\dot{V}\text{o}_2$ (15%)

thus reduced O_2 reserve and increased O_2 consumption emphasize importance of preoxygenation

Blood

- Increased intravascular fluid volume, maximum increase of 50% at 33–36 weeks
- Increase in red cell volume, but less so than the intravascular fluid volume increase resulting in dilutional anaemia
- Decreased viscosity ?
- Clotting diathesis (venous thrombosis is more common during and shortly after pregnancy)

CVS

- Increased heart rate, stroke volume and cardiac output (by 30–50%)
- Reduced peripheral resistance, reduced blood pressure
- Dilated skin vessels (warm skin, dilated veins)
- Liability to aortocaval compression (revealed and concealed)

Gastrointestinal system (GIS)

- Increased dental caries
- Gastric stasis
- Increased intragastric pressure
- Increased gastrin and acid production
- Liability to reflux in some subjects

Renal

- Increased glomerular filtration rate (GFR)
- Reduced renal glucose threshold may cause glycosuria
- Tendency to bacteriuria and urinary tract infection

Metabolic

- Increased basal metabolic rate (BMR)
- Reduced glucose tolerance
- Increased tendency to ketosis ('accelerated starvation state')
- Increased thyroid-binding globulin

CNS

- Reduced volume of epidural space (due to epidural venous distension; 30% less volume of anaesthetic required for same spread as in non-pregnant)

Placental flow varies with

- Maternal blood pressure
- Placental vascular tone

- Uterine contraction
- Placental pathology

Placental vascular tone is influenced by catecholamines (alpha receptors cause constriction) and hypocarbia (also constricts). Epidural may increase flow by relieving these factors.

GERIATRIC

Respiratory

- Reduced pulmonary elastic recoil (so airway closure occurs at a higher lung volume)
- Reduced FRC to less than closing volume (by the age of 65 years the FRC becomes less than the closing volume when standing; the situation is even worse in the supine posture)
- Increased (A–a) O_2 difference
- Increased dead space (V_D)
- Increased diaphragmatic respiration (in relation to intercostal)

CVS

- Decreased arterial compliance
- Decreased cardiac output
- Increased vein fragility

Metabolic

- Decreased BMR
- Defective temperature control (tendency to hypothermia)
- Reduced serum albumin

Renal

- Reduced GFR
- Liability to prostatism

CNS

- High incidence of postoperative cognitive deficit
- Increased sensitivity to central depressants
- Liability to central anticholinergic syndrome
- Deafness (impairs communication)
- Increased epidural spread of local agents

Neuromuscular

- Reduced muscle bulk

- Muscle weakness
- Mobilization problems

Immunology

- Decreased competence

General

- Frequent coexisting disease and medication

CENTRAL NERVOUS SYSTEM

NEUROSURGERY

- General condition of patient often poor (trauma, hypertension, ischaemic heart disease, diabetes)
- Raised intracranial pressure (must be avoided and reduced where already present)
- Avoid hypertensive response to intubation; consider:
  — Opioids – alfentanil
  — Lidocaine (lignocaine)
  — β-blocker – esmolol
  — Repeat dosage of induction agent prior to intubation
- Ensure full muscle relaxation prior to intubation
- Long operations
- Airway:
  — Inaccessible due to positioning and drapes
  — Need for free airway (no coughing and straining)
  — Reinforced endotracheal tube to prevent kinking
- Posture (sitting position may be associated with hypotension and high risk of air embolism)
- Need to allow adequate venous drainage (head up tilt, no extreme rotation of head)
- Need for rapid recovery so neurological signs can be evaluated soon after end of surgery

CONTROL OF INTRACRANIAL PRESSURE (ICP)

The skull is essentially of fixed volume so changes in the volume of the intracranial contents will result in pressure changes. The contents include brain tissue, cerebrospinal fluid (CSF), blood and interstitial fluid.

Methods of ICP control

With the exception of surgical CSF drainage and decompression, methods for control of ICP depend on reducing intracerebral blood volume or reducing interstitial fluid.

Intracerebral blood volume
- This may be reduced by cerebral vessel vasoconstriction (induced by control of P_aCO_2) and by lowering venous pressure. In cases where autoregulation is defective arterial blood pressure also requires control

Reduction of interstitial fluid
- This can be achieved by administration of diuretics. Agents frequently used include furosemide (frusemide) and mannitol. Mannitol will cause an expansion of the intravascular volume (with a rise of the central venous pressure and blood pressure); also passage of osmotically active agents into the brain substance (across a damaged blood–brain barrier) can retain fluid in the brain
- Steroids can also be used to reduce interstitial fluid. They are useful for discrete slow-growing lesions but ineffective when administered after trauma

Management of Raised Intracranial Pressure

- In all patients with raised intracranial pressure first-line management involves attention to general principles:
  — Maintenance of arterial oxygenation
  — Maintenance of cerebral perfusion pressure (70 mmHg or greater)
  — Complete volume resuscitation
  — Control of pyrexia
  — Control of seizures
  — Elevation of head of bed (to reduce cerebral venous pressure)
  — Avoidance of jugular venous obstruction
  — Sedation +/− paralysis
- The development of an intracranial mass lesion should always be suspected and excluded in patients with raised or increasing intracranial pressure
- With the exception of surgical CSF drainage and decompression, methods for control of ICP depend on reducing intracerebral blood volume or reducing interstitial fluid

First-line treatment of raised pressure (non-surgical)
- CSF drainage from intraventricular catheter (if in situ).
- Ventilation adjustment to achieve low eucapnia (P_aCO_2 4.5 kPa) – preferably with jugular venous oxygen saturation (S_jO_2) monitoring
- Mannitol (limited by a serum osmolality of 320 mOsm/l and with monitoring of fluid status to avoid hypovolaemia)

Second tier treatments (which appear to reduce ICP but have more risk or which have an unproven effect on outcome)
- Barbiturates
- Hypothermia
- Hyperventilation to a $P_a co_2$ of <4 kPa (with associated monitoring for cerebral ischaemia)
- Decompressive craniotomy

CEREBRAL BLOOD FLOW (CBF)

$$\text{Cerebral perfusion pressure (CPP)} = \text{mean arterial pressure (MAP)} - \text{intracranial pressure (ICP)}$$

Normal cerebral perfusion pressure = 80 mmHg
Critical cerebral perfusion pressure = 30 mmHg

CBF varies with

Arterial pressure
- Autoregulation between MAP of 60–160 mmHg, but takes 60–120 seconds to react so CBF becomes raised for this period. Autoregulation is disrupted by trauma, volatile anaesthetic agents, seizures and in the region of tumours

Venous pressure
- Venous pressure increased by: head-down posture, constriction of the neck, twisting of the neck, coughing, straining or struggling, raised intrathoracic pressure

$P_a co_2$
- Hypocarbia results in a reduced CBF (30% at $P_a co_2$ of 3.5 kPa)
- Hypercarbia results in an increased CBF (100% at $P_a co_2$ of 8–11 kPa). *N.B.* 90% return to baseline CBF 4 h after change of $P_a co_2$ and complete in 6–12 h (parallels CSF H^+ changes)

CSF pressure
$P_a o_2$
- Less influence on CBF than is the case with $P_a co_2$. Increase of CBF begins when $P_a o_2$ falls to 8 kPa

Special features

High blood flow = 50 ml min^{-1}/100 g
Critical flow = 18–24 ml min^{-1}/100 g
90% of flow via internal carotids (10% via vertebrals)

Steal
- Area of fixed vasodilation due to trauma or ischaemia will receive less blood flow when adjacent normal brain becomes vasodilated (e.g. in response to hypercapnia)

Reverse steal
- Area of fixed vasodilation due to trauma or ischaemia will receive more blood flow when adjacent normal brain becomes vasoconstricted (e.g. in response to hypocapnia)

HEAD INJURY

The general principles of head injury management are as follows:

Blood pressure and oxygenation goals after severe traumatic brain injury (TBI)

- Hypotension (systolic blood pressure < 60 mmHg) or hypoxia (cyanosis or P_aO_2 < 8 kPa) should be scrupulously avoided or corrected immediately (good evidence)
- MAP should be kept above 90 mmHg in an attempt to maintain the cerebral perfusion pressure (CPP) > 70 mmHg (probably valuable, unclear evidence)

Intracranial pressure (ICP) monitoring

- Patients with an abnormal CT scan and a Glasgow Coma Score (GCS) of <9 should have ICP monitored
- Patients with a normal CT scan but with two or more of the following should have their ICP monitored:
  — Abnormal motor posturing
  — Age > 40 years
  — Systolic blood pressure < 90 mmHg
- Normal ICP is 0–10 mmHg. Most clinicians would consider pressures in excess of 20 mmHg as an indication for treatment

Cerebral perfusion pressure

- Maintenance at a minimum of 70 mmHg is recommended

Hyperventilation

- In the absence of raised ICP, prolonged hyperventilation should now be avoided after severe TBI. There is good evidence that routine hyperventilation is detrimental.

- The use of prophylactic hyperventilation (P_aCO_2 <4.5 kPa) during the first 24 h after severe TBI (when CBF is known to be reduced) should be avoided
- Hyperventilation may be used for brief periods to reduce ICP during episodes of acute neurological deterioration. When hyperventilation is employed, monitoring of jugular venous oxygen saturation (S_jO_2) may identify resulting cerebral hypoxia (due to vasoconstriction as a consequence of the low P_aCO_2). N.B. The S_jO_2 should be >50%. Lower values suggest cerebral hypoxia

Mannitol

- Mannitol effectively reduces ICP at a dose of 0.25–1 g/kg

Barbiturates

- High dose barbiturate may usefully reduce ICP in haemodynamically stable patients with intractable raised ICP following severe TBI

Glucocorticoids

- Glucocorticoids are not recommended in the treatment of severe TBI (there is good evidence that they are not helpful)

Reference

Brain Trauma Foundation, American Association of Neurological Surgeons, Joint Section on Neurotrauma and Critical Care 1996 Guidelines for the management of severe head injury. Journal of Neurotrauma 13(11): 641–734

AIR EMBOLISM

During surgery air embolism can occur due to faulty intravenous technique (e.g. unprimed giving sets), disconnection of central venous lines where central venous pressure is low (Leur lock connections are advocated to connect to central venous lines) or opening of veins which are at sub-atmospheric pressure. The highest risk is in spontaneously breathing neurosurgical patients who are in the sitting position for surgery.

Major danger areas

- Mastoid emissary vein
- Suboccipital triangle
- Muscles in the back of the neck
- Diploë of the skull

Signs

- Respiratory disturbance (increased rate and irregularity)
- Tachycardia
- Hypotension
- Cyanosis
- Unconsciousness in unanaesthetized patients

Detection

- Close observation of clinical signs especially at times of risk during surgery
- Fall of end tidal CO_2
- Doppler ultrasound (very sensitive)
- Heart murmur ('mill wheel') detected by stethoscope (late and insensitive)
- S-T depression on the electrocardiogram
- Rise in pulmonary artery pressure (in proportion to volume of air)

Prevention

- Maintain a high CVP (unless contraindicated)
- Use of positive end expiratory pressure (PEEP)
- Use of antigravity suit

Management

- Immediate flooding of the wound with saline
- Immediate compression of the neck veins
- Stop N_2O, give 100% O_2
- Lower the head (to raise venous pressure)
- Place in left lateral position, if practical
- Attempt to aspirate air from CVP or pulmonary artery line where these are in situ

INTRACRANIAL ANEURYSM

- Patients are often young and fit, but may be hypertensive and dehydrated
- Hypertension must be avoided, particularly on tracheal intubation (or the aneurysm may rebleed)
- Hypotension will be required during surgery – requirement for fast onset and reversible lowering of blood pressure (BP)
- ICP must be maintained at low levels
- Straining and coughing must be avoided
- Air embolism is a risk

- Surgery may be prolonged
- Access to the patient and airway is restricted; monitoring is important
- Local arterial spasm may result in cerebral infarction
- Antifibrinolytic agents may have been given (with the object of reducing the incidence of rebleeding)
- Repeat anaesthesia likely (diagnostic angiography, surgery for clipping of the aneurysm, postoperative angiography)
- Massive blood loss is a possibility – high blood flow to brain $(50\,\mathrm{ml\,min^{-1}}/100\,\mathrm{g})$
- Cerebral protection – use of hypothermia, barbiturates or steroids may be indicated

CAROTID ENDARTERECTOMY

- Surgery of proven benefit if 70% stenosis
- Patients are often elderly with generalized arterial disease including coronary and vertebral arteries
- May be smokers, diabetic
- 70% hypertensive, and preoperative control improves morbidity

Maintain cerebral blood flow

During carotid occlusion blood flow to compromised hemisphere depends on collateral flow via the circle of Willis or the vertebral arteries.

- Avoid hypotension and extreme hypertension
- Induced hypertension – moderate increase advocated by some
- Carotid shunt controversial
- Hypercapnia thought ineffective (ischaemic areas may already be maximally dilated and hypercapnia may cause steal)
- Beware obstruction by extreme neck positions of atheromatous vertebral arteries in patients with cervical osteoarthritis; cerebral supply may depend on vertebral flow where carotids are stenosed

Cerebral protection

- Avoid hypoxia
- Barbiturate anaesthesia
- Use isoflurane
- Heparinization
- Maintain normoglycaemia
- Timing of surgery–clamp < 20 min if possible
- Avoid nitrous oxide
- Hypothermia (generally impractical)
- Consider carotid shunt during surgery

Monitoring

- Stump pressure (maintain > 50–60 mmHg)
- Cerebral function – electroencephalogram (EEG), somatosensory evoked potentials
- Jugular venous Po_2 (low values reflect low perfusion)
- Xenon clearance (complicated radioisotope study)
- Retinal plethysmography
- Observation of the patient during surgery under local anaesthesia

Postoperative problems

- Myocardial ischaemia
- Hypertension – consider control by intravenous agents
- Hypotension – treat hypovolaemia, consider sympathomimetics
- Haemorrhage from carotid – beware difficult intubation
- Neurological deficit (in up to 7%)

Reference

Garrioch M A, Fitch W 1993 Anaesthesia for carotid artery surgery. British Journal of Anaesthesia 71: 569–579

SPINAL ANAESTHESIA

Advantages

- Simple and quick to perform (vs epidural or nerve blocks)
- Rapid onset
- Profound analgesia
- Muscle relaxation
- Low dose so no systemic toxicity
- Reduced surgical haemorrhage
- Increased lower limb blood flow with a lower incidence of deep venous thrombosis (DVT)
- Laryngeal reflexes and consciousness preserved = less risk of pulmonary aspiration
- Predictable spread with hyperbaric solutions (more localization of block than is possible with epidural anaesthesia)
- Preserves visceral blood flow
- Use of opioids allows prolonged analgesia

Disadvantages

- Single shot – limited duration
- Hypotension
- Headache – post dural puncture headache

- Hearing disturbance
- Discomfort during needle insertion and positioning
- Meningitis
- Neurological sequelae:
  — Wrong solution injected
  — Contaminant
  — Needle trauma
  — Haematoma
  — Cord ischaemia secondary to hypotension
- Idiosyncrasy

Contraindications

Absolute
- Patient refusal
- Bleeding diathesis
- Sepsis (particularly of overlying back)
- Uncompensated fluid depletion
- Raised ICP

Relative
- Aortic stenosis
- Severe coronary artery disease or fixed cardiac output
- Severe back deformity/ankylosis
- Neurological disease
- Bowel perforation (unopposed vagal parasympathetic action with sympathetic blockade results in contraction of the bowel with possible increased peritoneal contamination)

Headache

The incidence of post dural puncture headache depends on the age of the patient (reduced incidence in those over 45), the type of needle being used, direction of orientation of the bevel and the sex of the patient when using larger Quincke needles.

Prevention
- With Quincke needle:
  — Use of small needle (26 G or smaller considerably reduces incidence)
  — Penetration of dura with bevel parallel to fibres
- Use of conical tip needle (e.g. Whitacre or Sprotte)
- Encouragement of fluid intake
- Avoidance of straining and upright posture after procedure

Treatment
- Analgesia

- Lying down, encourage fluid intake
- Abdominal binder/prone posture (increased intra-abdominal pressure distends epidural veins and limits CSF flow into the epidural space)
- Epidural drip with suitable crystalloid
- Epidural blood patch is the most effective treatment

Reference

Morgan P 1995 Spinal anaesthesia in obstetrics. Canadian Journal of Anaesthesia 42(12): 1145–1163

SPINAL INJURY MANAGEMENT

Initial stages

- Immobilization and maintenance of blood pressure (mean 65–70 mmHg is suggested minimum) and oxygenation to avoid extension of neurological damage
- The phrenic nerve emanates from C3/4/5. Early airway control is advisable where there is any doubt. Patients with cervical cord injury may initially maintain minute ventilation with intercostal muscles and abdominal breathing but eventually tire. They will then develop progressive respiratory failure or may rapidly suffer respiratory arrest. Orotracheal intubation with in-line cervical spine stabilization and cricoid pressure is generally considered to be the optimal intubation method in cervical spine injury. Gastric stasis is common following injury
- Hypotension in patients with spinal cord injury may be due to the cord injury or to blood loss from a concurrent injury (or a combination of both). Cervical or high thoracic cord injury results in sympathetic denervation, which results in vasodilation and bradycardia (patients with hypovolaemic shock but without spinal injury may also present with bradycardia, although tachycardia is characteristic)
- Priapism and loss of anal tone imply complete spinal cord injury
- Vasodilation associated with spinal shock and paralysis preventing effective shivering can rapidly result in significant hypothermia if preventive measures are not instituted
- Acute urinary retention is to be expected in cases of complete injury
- Pressure ulceration occurs very readily if not actively avoided
- Concomitant cervical spine injury has been identified in 8% of patients with a Glasgow Coma Score < 10
- Anteroposterior, lateral and odontoid X-ray views are required to evaluate the cervical spine (and must include views of the lower vertebrae). N.B. Prevertebral space anterior to C3 in excess of 5 mm suggests cervical spine injury
- A step of 3.7 mm or angulation > 11° on X-ray indicates instability of the spine

- National Acute Spinal Cord Injury Study (NASCIS) suggested that for patients with blunt spinal cord injury and neurological signs, methylprednisolone (30 mg/kg bolus then 5.4 mg/kg over 23 h) might reduce eventual neurological deficit. Must be given within 8 h of injury
- Cord lesions with progressive neurological signs require surgical intervention

Medium-term

- Adrenergic crisis (mass autonomic response in the denervated region in response to stimulation in this area)
- DVT
- Hyperkalaemic response to suxamethonium (should be avoided as cardiac arrest may occur 3 days–12 months post-injury)
- Cervical spine fixation may cause intubation difficulties

Long-term

- Contractures
- Sepsis (particularly of urinary tract)
- Renal failure (now rare)
- Psychological disturbance

Reference

Baron B J, Scalea T M 2000 Spinal Cord Injuries. In: Tintinalli J E, Kelen G D, Stapczynski J S, eds. Emergency medicine: a comprehensive study guide, 5th edition. McGraw-Hill, New York, ch 248, pp 1645–1660

ENDOTRACHEAL INTUBATION

Advantages

- Avoids airway obstruction (with straining, hypercarbia and hypoxia)
- Facilitates intermittent positive pressure ventilation (IPPV)
- Protects the airway from soiling (cuffed tube)
- Permits surgical access to the head and neck
- Reduces dead space
- Direct access for sputum aspiration

Disadvantages

- Trauma during intubation
- Deeper anaesthesia may be required to permit intubation and toleration of endotracheal tube

- Muscle relaxant may be required to facilitate endotracheal intubation
- Sympathetic response to laryngoscopy, intubation and extubation may be hazardous (e.g. in coronary artery disease or cerebral aneurysm)
- Bypasses the nasal–oral warming and humidification mechanism
- Instrumentation of the trachea introduces and encourages infection
- Failed intubation or unrecognized oesophageal intubation is hazardous, especially in patients to whom muscle relaxants have been administered
- Respiratory obstruction can still occur should the endotracheal tube become occluded
- Sub-glottic oedema and stenosis can be a complication, especially in long-term intubation and in children

DIFFICULT INTUBATION

Grading (by view at laryngoscopy)

Grade 1   Most of glottis visible
Grade 2   Only posterior aspect of glottis is visible (cuneiform, corniculate cartilages)
Grade 3   No part of glottis visible, epiglottis can be seen
Grade 4   Hard palate only visible (epiglottis not seen)

Incidence

- About 1% found to be Grade 3 or 4
- 20% not predictable

Features suggesting intubation difficulty

- Restricted mouth opening (scar, scleroderma, temporomandibular joint ankylosis, indurated infection, etc.)
- Receding mandible
- Prominent or isolated teeth
- Swelling at base of mouth
- High, arched palate
- Short, immobile neck
- Laryngeal pathology
- Stridor
- Epiglottitis
- Congenital problems – Pierre Robin's, Turner's and Treacher Collins' syndromes

Scoring systems

- Mallampati – problem with specificity of test, too many false positives:

Class	Structures visible
I	Soft palate, fauces, pillars and uvula
II	Soft palate, fauces and uvula
III	Soft palate, base of uvula only
IV	Hard palate only (this added in modified Mallampati system)

- Improve specificity if combine Class IV with one of the following (improve further with two):
  — Receding chin
  — Short neck
  — Protruding maxillary incisors

Useful equipment for potential intubation difficulty (Fig. 1.1)

- Various laryngoscope blades, such as Magill, McCoy and Polio
- Fibreoptic intubating laryngoscope
- Various endotracheal tubes (including small lumen tubes)
- Variety of oral and nasal airways
- Laryngeal mask, intubating laryngeal mask
- Introducers and gum elastic bougie
- Cricothyroid needle or 'minitrach'
- Emergency tracheostomy equipment
- Also, experienced assistance should be on hand and in some cases a surgeon should be alerted to the possibility that tracheostomy may be required (epiglottitis, laryngeal tumours)

References

Cormack R S, Lethane J 1984 Difficult tracheal intubation in obstetrics. Anaesthesia 39: 1105–1111
Cobley M, Vaughan R S 1992 Recognition and management of difficult airway problems. British Journal of Anaesthesia 68: 90–97

GASTRIC ACID ASPIRATION PREVENTION

Aim

To keep gastric fluid pH > 3.0, volume < 25 ml and to prevent regurgitation or vomiting, especially when laryngeal reflexes are compromised.

Risk population

- Unfasted patients
- Obstetric patients:
  — Delayed emptying due to altered stomach position, gastric hypotonia and opioids during labour
  — Increased acid secretion

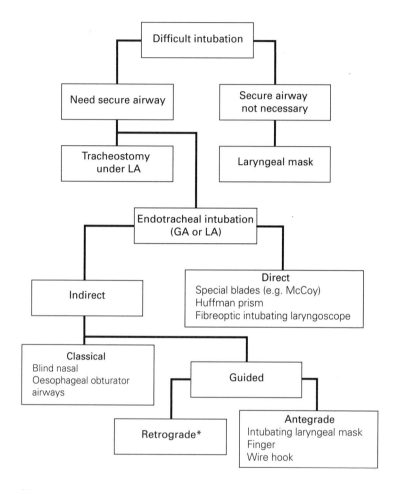

GA – general anaesthesia; LA – local anaesthetic

* Water's technique – passage of an epidural catheter through the cricothyroid membrane and into the oropharynx via the larynx. The catheter is then pulled through the nose to be used as a guide for the passage of a nasal tube.

Fig. 1.1

- Patients with bowel obstruction (especially upper)
- Patients with ileus
- Diabetic patients (autonomic neuropathy with gastric stasis)
- Renal failure patients (high gastrin levels)
- Obese patients
- Those with a history of oesophageal reflux
- Patients with an intra-abdominal mass

Manipulations

Reduction of gastric acid production
- Anticholinergics unreliable
- H_2-receptor antagonists reduce acidity and volume of gastric fluid

Neutralization of gastric acid
- Magnesium trisilicate BPC:
  — Must be freshly prepared
  — May not mix well (aided by rotation of patient)
  — Is particulate (may cause pulmonary damage in its own right if aspirated)
  — May layer and is unpalatable
- Sodium citrate (0.3 molar):
  — Is stable
  — Mixes more reliably
  — Is non-particulate
  — Only reliably neutralizes gastric acid for 45 min after administration

Gastric emptying
- Nasogastric or orogastric tube (unpleasant and may not totally empty stomach; double-lumen 'sump' type tubes are more effective)
- Apomorphine induction of vomiting (may be unpleasant for patient; severe autonomic effects may be associated)
- Metoclopramide promotes gastric emptying into the duodenum and small bowel (antagonized by atropine and opioids)

Increase of lower oesophageal sphincter (LOS) tone
The lower oesophageal sphincter tone – intragastric pressure is referred to as the 'barrier pressure'

- Metoclopramide, suxamethonium and pancuronium have been shown to increase LOS tone (however, prior anticholinergic or opioid therapy may inhibit the action of metoclopramide)

Prevention of passive reflux of gastric fluid into oropharynx and trachea should it pass the LOS and enter the oesophagus
- Occlusion of the upper oesophagus by pressure on the cricoid cartilage (Sellick's manoeuvre)
- Positioning of patients at risk (including during the recovery period) in a head-down lateral position

Important general factors

- The stomach should be emptied if possible
- Equipment should be checked; in particular high volume suction equipment must be available
- The table on which the patient is to be induced must tip head down

- Careful pre-oxygenation should be given
- Trained assistance is important, especially for the performance of effective cricoid pressure
- Knowledge of 'failed intubation drill' is important for both anaesthetist and assistants

FAILED INTUBATION DRILL

- Developed for obstetric practice, introduced by Tunstall in 1976
- Important for all emergency anaesthesia

In the event of finding it impossible to intubate patient:

- Do not persist in attempt to intubate (this includes attempts by other anaesthetists)
- Mobilize help from colleagues in theatre, one to phone for senior assistance
- Maintain cricoid pressure (assistant should use both hands)
- Oxygenate patient by utilizing all means at your disposal – initially try with bag and mask, add airway, use both hands to maintain airway and allow someone else to squeeze reservoir bag, remove cricoid pressure and consider laryngeal mask if necessary
- If impossible to oxygenate use transtracheal injection technique

Once patient is oxygenated and spontaneous ventilation returns, turn patient onto left lateral position and assess urgency of procedure to be performed.

- If not life threatening wake patient up, carefully explain the situation to the patient and perform under regional block with senior assistance
- If impossible to perform operation under regional block or condition life threatening:
  — Introduce volatile anaesthetic and breathe patient down to surgical anaesthesia
  — Introduce laryngeal mask, position patient and proceed (under spontaneous respiration)

Reference

Harmer M 1997 Difficult and failed intubation in obstetrics. International Journal of Obstetric Anaesthesia 6: 25–31

MANAGEMENT OF ASPIRATION

Incidence reported between 1:2000–14000 anaesthetics with mortality 1:70000–140000.

- Aspiration may lead to pneumonitis

- Risk and severity related to volume, pH and other factors (not yet known)
- If severe leads to:
  Stage 1 (immediate tissue injury, potential airway blockage with food)
  — Breath holding
  — Coughing
  — Severe bronchospasm
  — Cyanosis
  Stage 2 (inflammatory response)
  — Neutrophil response to cytokines released
  — Massive shift of circulating fluid into pulmonary interstitium causing circulatory collapse and gas exchange problems
  — Bacterial infection

Treatment

- Oxygen
- Intubation desirable – facilitates bronchial suction, oxygen therapy and IPPV when necessary
- Vascular access – infuse plasma expander
- Instillation of small volumes of normal saline may facilitate bronchial suction (*N.B.* initial acid load dispersed quickly in lungs)
- Treat bronchospasm with nebulized salbutamol and/or intravenous aminophylline
- Maintain oxygenation – use IPPV and PEEP as indicated
- Maintain circulation – monitor CVP, urine output
- Antibiotics – as per local antibiotic policy (mainly consider anaerobes)

Reference

Engelhardt T, Webster N R 1999 Pulmonary aspiration of gastric contents in anaesthesia. British Journal of Anaesthesia 83: 453–460

COEXISTING DISEASE

PYLORIC STENOSIS

- Low weight, usually 2–6-week-old males
- May have hypochloraemic hypokalaemic alkalosis with dehydration which should be corrected preoperatively
- May have paradoxical aciduria when dehydration is severe. Need to conserve Na^+ overrides need to conserve H^+, therefore renal Na^+/H^+ exchange

- There is potentially a full stomach, even hours after a feed. Should be aspirated, gastric washout should be performed preoperatively and precautions taken to prevent aspiration
- Hypoglycaemia can occur with preoperative starvation
- Heat loss is significant in these small children unless precautions are taken
- Postoperative respiratory monitoring is important as apnoea is common

CYSTIC FIBROSIS

- Commonest fatal inherited disease of Caucasians, incidence of $1:2000$ births
- Gene carried by 5% of the population
- Exocrine abnormality with recessive mode of inheritance
- 80% of sufferers reach adulthood with median life expectancy of 40 years

Clinical features

Respiratory
- Repeated infections leading to bronchiectasis
- Progressive mixed obstructive/restrictive defect
- Terminal respiratory failure with cysts (honeycombing) and fibrosis on chest X-ray and cor pulmonale
- Pneumothorax occurs in 20% of adults
- Nasal polyps common
- Elevated $P_a\text{co}_2$ indicates severe disease

Gastrointestinal
- Meconium ileus – presenting feature in 15% of patients
- Rectal prolapse – in 20% of children
- Pancreatic fibrosis and insufficiency (malabsorption, occasionally diabetes)
- Biliary cirrhosis

Sweat deficiency
- May become hyperthermic, especially in tropical environments

Diagnosis

The diagnosis is confirmed by a sweat test (high Na^+ content).

Anaesthetic considerations

- Sputum retention (tenacious sputum)
- Hypoxia ($\dot{V}/\dot{Q}$ abnormality)
- Bronchial hyperreactivity (liability to bronchospasm)

- Emphysematous bullae may rupture with IPPV
- Possible nasal obstruction
- Malabsorption (vitamin K deficiency may result in clotting factor deficiency and increased bleeding; may be less albumin for drug binding)
- Possible diabetes

Management

- Preoperative lung function, chest X-ray (CXR) and blood glucose tests
- Intensive preoperative physiotherapy; sputum culture and antibiotic where indicated
- ECG, echocardiography, arterial blood gases (ABGs) and coagulation screen when indicated
- Good preoxygenation
- Good hydration/humidification
- Generally best with regional technique or intubation with ventilation
- Beware risk of pneumothorax or pulmonary collapse
- Intensive postoperative physiotherapy; regional postoperative analgesia preferable

Reference

Walsh T S, Young C H 1995 Anaesthesia and cystic fibrosis. Anaesthesia 50: 614–622

RENAL DISEASE/TRANSPLANTATION

- Electrolyte disturbance (particularly hyperkalaemia)
- Acidosis, uraemia
- Fluid imbalance (overhydration or dehydration)
- Hypertension common (though Na^+ depletion and hypotension can also occur)
- Anaemia (but increased red cell 2,3-DPG and acidosis result in a right shift of the oxyhaemoglobin dissociation curve)
- Reduced renal drug excretion (action of gallamine especially prolonged)
- May be hypoalbuminaemic (nephrotic syndrome)
- Patients may have neuropathy
- Commonly poor veins; shunts should be avoided for the injection of anaesthetic drugs which may thrombose them
- Patients frequently on drug treatment (steroids, hypotensives, diuretics)
- May have red cell antibodies following previous transfusions
- May have HBsAg
- Gastric hyperacidity
- Patients may be unprepared for anaesthesia especially in cases for renal transplant

- Liability to infection (due to effects of renal failure and subsequent immunosuppressant therapy after transplant)
- In patients with renal failure beware sevoflurane, methoxyflurane (potential renal toxicity) and suxamethonium (risk of hyperkalaemia)
- Maintenance of BP to ensure patency of shunts and perfusion of transplanted kidney

LIVER DISEASE

- Causes toxicity, autoimmune disease and viral infections
- Need to consider cause and potential associated problems:
  - *Alcohol*: consider cardiomyopathy, poor nutrition and withdrawal
  - *Sclerosing cholangitis*: consider inflammatory bowel disease, preserved hepatic function until late in disease
  - *Primary biliary cirrhosis*: portal hypertension, hypersplenism and thrombocytopenia
- Reduced clotting factors: prothrombin, VII, IX and X (malabsorption of vitamin K in biliary obstruction, reduced synthesis in hepatocellular disease)
- Hypoglycaemia
- Hypoalbuminaemia
- Reduced intravascular volume
- Electrolyte disturbance
- Hypoxia (hepatopulmonary syndrome)
- Pleural effusions and may have ascites
- High incidence of gastro-oesophageal reflux
- Hyperbilirubinaemia (appears, in the presence of hypovolaemia, to predispose to renal tubular necrosis)
- Patients may carry the HbsAg, or be hepatitis C positive – danger to personel
- Anaesthesia can lead to fatal decompensation even if patient's condition stable
  - Result of reduced hepatic blood flow (due to IPPV), reduced cardiac output (CO) and BP, attenuation of the hepatic buffer response
- Viral hepatitis is a contraindication to anaesthesia as hepatic failure may follow
- Reduced drug metabolism
- Sensitivity to cerebral depressants; liable to encephalopathy
- Potential for raised ICP – beware volatile agents
- Patient assessment by risk factors has been suggested, factors include: bilirubin level, prothrombin time and grade of encephalopathy

Reference

Clarke P, Bellamy M C 2000 Anaesthesia for patients with liver disease. Bulletin 4. Royal College of Anaesthetists, pp 158–161

RHEUMATOID ARTHRITIS

Found in 3% of female and 1% of male population.
* Joint disease leads to difficulty with:
  — Patient positioning
  — Access for iv canulation (also have poor veins)
  — Access for regional techniques
* Intubation problems (restricted cervical spine mobility, temporomandibular joint ankylosis, crico-arytenoid involvement)
* Up to 30% may have cervical spine instability:
  — Ask about referred pain
  — Cervical spine X-ray mandatory (see page 187)
* May have cardiac involvement (pericarditis, amyloid, conduction defects and valve damage)
* Anaemia (secondary to chronic disease or due to GI blood loss associated with the use of NSAIDs)
* Neuropathy (distal symmetrical mixed, entrapment, mononeuritis multiplex – latter a bad prognostic sign)
* Lung involvement (fibrosis, effusion, nodules including Caplan's and bronchiectasis)
* Vasculitis, nodules (both associated with seropositivity)
* Sjögren's syndrome (dry eyes, mouth, bronchial tree)
* Felty's syndrome (hypersplenism, vasculitis)
* Drugs (anti-inflammatories cause bleeding; gold and penicillamine can cause blood dyscrasias, nephrotic syndrome and rashes; patients may also be taking steroids and cytotoxic agents)
* Amyloid and renal failure can complicate long-standing disease

Reference

Skues M A, Welchew E A 1993 Anaesthesia and rheumatoid arthritis. Anaesthesia 48: 989–997

ANKYLOSING SPONDYLITIS

* Cervical spine fusion and intubation difficulty
* Joint disease and difficulty positioning (particularly hip involvement and lithotomy)
* Restricted lung expansion; pulmonary fibrosis
* Aortic regurgitation
* Anaemia
* Uveitis
* Drug effects (particularly the gastric effects of anti-inflammatories)

OBESITY

Excessive body fat, body mass index (BMI) > 30 obese, > 35 morbidly obese.

* Increased morbidity and mortality when BMI > 30

- Difficult intubation (about 13% of cases)
- Reduced FRC, reduced vital capacity, reduced compliance
- Closing volume frequently exceeds FRC:
  — Resulting in $\dot{V}/\dot{Q}$ abnormality
  — Increased (a–a) O_2 difference (especially when supine)
  — Compounded by anaesthesia where FRC can be reduced by 50%
- Hypercapnia is rare but can occur in association with somnolence (termed 'pickwickian syndrome' after Joe in *The Pickwick Papers*)
- Airway difficulty (obstructive sleep apnoea link to difficult bag and mask ventilation)
- Predominant diaphragmatic respiration (vs intercostal respiration)
- Increased cardiac output; LVH
- Increased coronary artery disease
- Hypertension (usually mild or moderate, severe in 5–10%)
- Difficulty monitoring intraoperative blood pressure:
  — Non-invasive monitoring: cuff must be of appropriate size (large arms in obesity require large cuffs for accurate readings)
  — Consider arterial monitoring in most operations
- Gastric stasis (large gastric volumes) – use H_2 receptor antagonist (ranitidine) and prokinetic (metoclopramide) 12 h and 2 h before surgery
- Difficult venous access
- Problems with regional anaesthesia – but considered ideal, reduced epidural and spinal dose requirement
- Problems with positioning and mobilization:
  — Anaesthetize in theatre on appropriately rated operating table(s)
  — Beware pressure areas and neuropraxia
  — Beware inferior vena cava (IVC) compression
- Prolonged surgery
- Higher incidence of infection and of DVT
- Frequent association with type 2 diabetes (> 10%)
- Body water low (calculated as a proportion of total weight)
- Large depot of lipid-soluble agents
- Consider epidural infusion or patient controlled analgesia (PCA) for postoperative analgesia

Reference

Adams J P, Murphy P G 2000 Obesity in anaesthesia and intensive care. British Journal of Anaesthesia 85: 91–108

ALCOHOL

- Sedation
- Reduced cooperation; difficult neurological assessment
- Full stomach

- Emetic effect of alcohol
- Reduced laryngeal reflexes and airway control
- Hypothermia
- Decreased ability to compensate for haemorrhage
- Reduced antidiuretic hormone (ADH) secretion with resulting dehydration
- Delayed hypoglycaemia (particularly in children)
- Increased incidence of infection (especially bacterial pneumonias)

Additional effects of long-term consumption include

- Hepatic enzyme induction, liver dysfunction (hepatitis, cirrhosis)
- Tolerance to anaesthetic agents
- Neuropathy; cardiomyopathy
- Withdrawal effects (delirium tremens, convulsions, psychosis)
- Vitamin deficiencies – Korsakoff's, Wernicke's syndromes with:
  — Ophthalmoplegia
  — Nystagmus
  — Ataxia
  — Confusion
  — Amnesia with confabulation

DIABETES MELLITUS

Disease due to a relative or absolute deficiency of insulin ± insulin resistance leading to overproduction of glucose in the liver.

Features include

- Hyperglycaemia; glycosuria
- Hyperlipidaemia
- Microangiopathy (including neuropathy, renal failure)
- Atheroma
- Susceptibility to infection
- Hypoglycaemia
- Ketoacidosis, hyperosmolar coma

Two reasonably distinct types

Type I Pancreatic-cell destruction ketosis prone (previously 'juvenile', insulin dependent)

Type II Defective insulin secretion ± insulin resistance, non-ketosis prone (previously 'maturity onset', non-insulin dependent)

Biochemical effects of insulin include

- Enhancement of glycogen synthesis
- Increased conversion of glucose to fatty acid

- Facilitation of glucose transport across cell walls
- Inhibition of glycolysis, gluconeogenesis, lipolysis, glycogenolysis and ketogenesis
- Facilitation of K^+ transport into cells

Anaesthetic considerations

- Avoid hypoglycaemia (glucose administration as indicated)
- Avoid ketosis (insulin administration as indicated)
- Ensure good control of blood sugar; exclude ketoacidosis. These may be impossible where surgical problem destabilizes diabetes and compromise may be necessary:
  — Haemoglobin A_{Ic} concentration < 7% – good contol
  — Haemoglobin A_{Ic} concentration > 9% – poor contol, osmotic diuresis with water and electrolyte disturbance
  — Haemoglobin A_{Ic} concentration > 12% – verge of ketoacidosis
- Patients should be early on operating list if possible (not as important if on insulin infusion)
- Establish insulin infusion early in type 1 and those type 2 patients undergoing major surgery. Consider glucose–insulin–potassium (GIK) system or separate infusions of glucose and insulin
- Blood sugar should be measured in theatre
- Associated coronary, cerebral, renal and peripheral arterial disease
- Neuropathy (especially autonomic possible bradycardia, postural hypotension, reduced gastric emptying)
- Impaired renal function – important to maintain renal blood flow
- Reduced epidural dose requirement
- May have an effect on baricity of spinal agents
- Oral hypoglycaemic drugs should be discontinued the night before surgery (remember the prolonged action of chlorpropamide)

References

Sonksen P, Sonksen J 2000 Insulin: understanding its action in health and disease. British Journal of Anaesthesia 85: 69–79
McAnulty G R, Robertshaw H J, Hall G M 2000 Anaesthetic management of patients with diabetes mellitus. British Journal of Anaesthesia 85: 80–90

THYROIDECTOMY

- The airway may be obstructed by the goitre – intubation difficult in 6%
- May have endocrine disease, particularly thyrotoxicosis (affects 2% of women and 0.2% of men):
  — Symptoms – hyperactivity, weight loss and tremor
  — This should be controlled preoperatively as it increases BMR and $\dot{V}o_2$ – predisposes to congestive cardiac failure (CCF) and atrial fibrillation (AF) and can result in thyroid crisis ('storm')

- Control with carbimazole, propylthiouracil and β-blockers (6–8 weeks)
- Patients with hypothyroidism are very sensitive to central depressants, prone to CCF and excrete water and Na^+ loads poorly
- Exophthalmos of Graves' disease may be present; eyes must be protected during surgery
- Access to the airway is limited during surgery (armoured tube may be indicated)
- The goitre may extend retrosternally, necessitating thoracic surgery
- Bleeding may be profuse (minimized by preoperative iodine treatment to reduce gland vascularity)
- May require hypotensive techniques
- Patients may be on medication, particularly beta-blockers and thioureas (these can cause blood dyscrasias)
- Laryngeal damage may occur:
  - Bilateral superior laryngeal nerve damage causes severe stridor (abductors affected more than adductors – Semon's law)
  - Complete recurrent laryngeal nerve section causes cords to lie in mid-position and is not associated with stridor
- Postoperative bleeding into the neck can cause respiratory obstruction:
  - Important to realize need to release both skin and muscle stitches to release blood
- Parathyroid excision/damage may lead to postoperative hypoparathyroidism (and hypocalcaemia)

Reference

Farling P A 2000 Thyroid disease. British Journal of Anaesthesia 85: 15–28

PHAEOCHROMOCYTOMA

- Rare tumour arising from chromaffin cells in the adrenal medulla or in other sympathetic paraganglia (10% bilateral, 10% malignant)
- Hypertension (often paroxysmal), flush, sweating, hyperglycaemia, reduced plasma volume, increased haematocrit
- Diagnosis by measuring urinary free catecholamines in 24 h sample. Tumour location by computed axial tomography (CAT)/magnetic resonance imaging (MRI), venous sampling and radioimmunoassay of noradrenaline (norepinephrine)
- Associated with neurofibromatosis
- Preoperatively patients require alpha-adrenergic blockade (phenoxybenzamine is sedative) and concurrent intravascular fluid replacement. Beta-adrenergic blockade may be given in addition (should not be given before alpha-adrenergic blockade since this can precipitate severe hypertension and cardiac failure). Use of selective α_1 antagonists may reduce need for fluid replacement and use of β-blockers:

— Phenoxybenzamine – non specific α antagonist (non-competitive due to covalent binding to receptor)
— Prazosin – selective α_1 antagonist, has short half life
— Doxazosin – selective α_1 antagonist, long half life allowing once daily dosing

- Perioperative hypertension must be avoided (particularly during tracheal intubation, positioning and mobilization of the tumour):
  — Consider phentolamine/labetalol
- Histamine also causes noradrenaline (norepinephrine) release, hence histamine-releasing drugs should be avoided
- Perioperative hypotension may require:
  — Noradrenaline (norepinephrine) infusion
  — Other inotropes (methoxamine, phenylephrine)
  — Fluid
- Undiagnosed phaeochromocytoma for concurrent surgery is associated with high mortality

Reference

Prys-Roberts C 2000 Phaeochromocytoma – recent progress in its management. British Journal of Anaesthesia 85: 44–57

MYASTHENIA

Neuromuscular disease characterized by defective neuromuscular transmission with muscle weakness and excess fatiguability.

- May be associated thymoma (15% of cases), thyrotoxicosis or collagen disease
- Particularly affects middle-aged women
- Patients are sensitive to non-depolarizing neuromuscular blocking agents and are prone to develop 'dual' block with depolarizing drugs
- Anticholinesterase medication (usually pyridostigmine) omitted 4 h preoperatively while patients are closely observed for muscle weakness and respiratory sufficiency
- Endotracheal intubation is ideally achieved without relaxant. Where necessary, minimal doses of relaxant are required (titrated against clinical response)
- Postoperatively anticholinesterase drugs are reinstituted. Respiratory function must be closely monitored
- Chest infection is a serious risk, particularly following thoracotomy for thymectomy
- Overdose of anticholinesterase results in weakness due to cholinergic crisis
- Lack of response to intravenous edrophonium (anticholinesterase) differentiates this from myasthenic weakness

- Cholinergic crises is treated by pralidoxime (cholinesterase reactivator) and atropine, or by anticholinesterase withdrawal and respiratory support
- Eaton–Lambert syndrome – muscle weakness in patient with carcinoma (notably of bronchus). Differs in that it affects peripheral muscles more and shows little response to anticholinesterase drugs. Guanidine and calcium may have therapeutic value

Reference

Baraka A 1992 Anesthesia and myasthenia gravis. Canadian Journal of Anaesthesia 39: 476–486

MYOTONIA DYSTROPHICA

Autosomal dominant inheritance.

Progressive muscle disease characterized by wasting and inability to relax muscles. The electromyograph (EMG) shows characteristic repetition after discharges.

Other clinical features

- Characteristic blank facies and ptosis
- Frontal balding
- Cataracts
- Cardiomyopathy
- Cardiac conduction defects and tachyarrhythmias
- Disordered oesophageal mobility
- Endocrine deficiencies
- Gonadal atrophy
- Intellectual impairment

Anaesthetic considerations

- Muscle weakness, postoperative respiratory insufficiency and pulmonary complications common (sensitive to the effects of respiratory depressant drugs)
- Risk of aspiration (weakness and disordered oesophageal function)
- Masseter spasm (especially following suxamethonium administration). Spasm can also occur spontaneously; it is intrinsic to the muscle so neuromuscular blockade will not relieve it. Dantrolene appears ineffective
- Cardiomyopathy (sensitive to cardiac depressants)
- Risk of dysrhythmia or heart block
- Aggravated by cold (institute warming)
- Muscle spasms can be induced by hypoglycaemia
- Association with malignant hyperpyrexia

EPIGLOTTITIS

A severe bacterial throat infection with rapidly progressive inflammatory swelling of the epiglottis and supraglottis resulting in respiratory obstruction.

Previously most common in children in whom the organism was usually type B *Haemophilus influenzae* (more varied organisms in adults), but Hib vaccination has dramatically reduced the incidence in young children.

Clinical features

- Short history
- Progressive, severe sore throat
- Toxaemia; pyrexia
- Increasing dysphagia (salivary drooling)
- Stridor, respiratory distress
- Characteristic posture (sitting upright, neck extended)
- Usually, patients do not have harsh cough characteristic of tracheolaryngobronchitis (croup)

Differential diagnosis

- Tracheolaryngobronchitis
- Retropharyngeal abscess
- Foreign body
- Laryngeal diphtheria
- Infectious mononucleosis

Diagnostic tests

- Lateral neck X-ray
- Epiglottic swab
- Blood culture

(These tests should not be performed before the airway is secured)

Management

- Importance of hospital policy of care (? direct admission to intensive care unit (ICU))
- Reassure and avoid upsetting child (do not remove from parents)
- Keep upright (lying the patient down may provoke complete obstruction)
- Give O_2
- Consider nebulized adrenaline (epinephrine) and/or steroid

- Do not instrument the throat (attempted swabbing or indirect laryngoscopy can precipitate complete obstruction)
- Perform tracheal intubation (the swelling is supraglottic and the larynx is usually of normal calibre so smaller endotracheal tubes are not usually required)
- Intubation is usually only required for 24–48 h while swelling resolves following antibiotic treatment
- Antibiotic (usually third generation cephalosporin)

Intubation technique

- All equipment for difficult intubation present (various laryngoscope blades, a range of sizes and lengths of endotracheal tube, gum elastic bougies, tracheal tube introducers, cricothyroid needle, rigid bronchoscope)
- Skilled assistance
- Surgeon experienced in tracheostomy prepared with the necessary equipment
- Intravenous access (highly desirable but possibly unwise where this will provoke crying in small children)
- Emergency drugs at hand
- Monitoring prior to induction (pulse, blood pressure, ECG), providing this does not cause undue distress
- Calm inhalational induction in the sitting position
- Use of PEEP by pinching tail of reservoir bag can be useful
- Gentle direct laryngoscopy when satisfactory anaesthetic depth achieved
- Lifting of the epiglottis generally improves the airway; an orotracheal tube should be passed. Nasotracheal tube can be substituted when orotracheal intubation proves easy
- Spontaneous ventilation is usually satisfactory and most children require minimal sedation. Elbows should be splinted to prevent self-extubation
- Intubation should be continued for 24–48 h. Extubation should be performed where there are full facilities for anaesthesia and reintubation

MALIGNANT HYPERPYREXIA

- Inherited disorder of skeletal muscle with mortality of about 5%
- Characterized by attacks of excessive unrelieved muscle action thought to be related to defective sarcoplasmic binding of Ca^{2+} with resulting high muscle calcium levels
- Triggered by various factors, most importantly anaesthetic drugs
- First clear description by Denbrough from Australia in 1960
- Disease with similarities occurs in Landrace pigs

Incidence

1:50000 to 1:100000 anaesthetics (more frequent in paediatric practice, 1:15000).

Clinical features

- Masseter spasm following the use of suxamethonium
- Hypermetabolism:
  — Raised P_aco_2 –increasing $ETCO_2$
  — Tachypnoea (in unventilated patients)
  — Tachycardia
  — Reduced S_aO_2 (O_2 delivery unable to meet demands)
- Raised temperature (> 2°C per h, progressive)
- Muscle rigidity – generalized late onset rigidity is a sign of severe problems

Biochemical features

- Metabolic acidosis
- Increased serum potassium concentration
- Increased serum levels of muscle enzymes (creatinine phosphokinase (CPK), lactate dehydrogenase (LDH), serum glutamic-oxaloacetic transaminase (SGOT))
- Myoglobinaemia (renal failure can ensue)

Treatment

- Stop all volatiles
- Hyperventilate on 100% O_2 (preferably using circuit unexposed to volatile agent)
- Maintain anaesthesia with intravenous drugs
- Stop surgery as soon as possible
- Active cooling measures but avoid overzealous application of ice leading to vasoconstriction
- Reconstitute dantrolene and give each 20 mg bottle as it becomes available until clinical signs start to subside – average dose 3 mg/kg but up to 10 mg/kg needed
- Monitor temperature, pulse, ECG
- Check blood gases and electrolytes
- Treat acidosis and hyperkalaemia (bicarbonate and dextrose/insulin as indicated)
- Maintain diuresis

Testing

(both patient and blood relatives of identified cases)

- In vitro muscle contraction – susceptible muscle contracts in response to halothane, caffeine and ryanodine exposure
- Serum CPK levels (unreliable, as normal in 60% of those susceptible)

Incriminated drugs

- Suxamethonium
- Volatile agents
- Phenothiazines – less certain but easily avoided in anaesthesia
- Atropine (said to make attack more fulminant, but not a trigger agent)

Drugs which appear safe

- Propofol, thiopental and etomidate
- Fentanyl
- Non-depolarizing muscle relaxants (avoid tubocurare)
- Prilocaine, bupivacaine and lidocaine (lignocaine)
- Diazepam

References

Denbrough M A, Lovell R R H 1960 Anaesthetic deaths in a family. Lancet ii: 45
Hopkins P M 2000 Malignant hyperthermia: advances in clinical management and diagnosis. British Journal of Anaesthesia 85: 118–128

PLASMA CHOLINESTERASE VARIANTS

Enzyme responsible for the breakdown of suxamethonium by hydrolysis: suxamethonium → succinylmonocholine → succinic acid + choline

Prolonged suxamethonium activity can be due to

- Decreased plasma cholinesterase levels
- Inhibition of plasma cholinesterase activity
- Abnormal cholinesterase

Decreased plasma cholinesterase

- Reduction of normal plasma cholinesterase by 30% has minimal effect
- Produced by the liver so may be reduced in liver disease, and malnutrition
- Removed by plasmapheresis
- Low levels of enzyme have been noted during pregnancy, maximal at 2–3 days post delivery, rarely of clinical significance except in heterozygotes

Inhibition of cholinesterase enzyme activity

Noncompetitive
- Organophosphates (pesticides or ecothiopate eye-drops)
- Cyclophosphamide reduces activity by up to 50%

Competitive
- Tetrahydroaminoacridine (anticholinesterase that was used to prolong suxamethonium action, others, e.g. neostigmine, also extend action)
- Propanidid, pancuronium and metoclopramide have been shown to inhibit plasma cholinesterase

Abnormal cholinesterase

- There are a number of genetically determined types of abnormal enzyme which result in a prolonged action of suxamethonium. The enzyme is determined by alleles found on the long arm of chromosome 3, some of which are termed:
  — Usual (normal)   U
  — Dibucaine resistant ('atypical') A
  — Fluoride resistant   F
  — Silent   S
  However the silent gene may consist of several different alleles and further variants have now been identified.

Abnormal enzymes can be differentiated by their resistance to inhibition of hydrolytic activity by dibucaine or fluoride in vitro (normal cholinesterase is inhibited).
  Many genotypes are possible which are associated with different suxamethonium sensitivity (see Table 1.3).

Table 1.3 Suxamethonium sensitivity

	% inhibition			
	Dibucaine	Fluoride	Incidence	Sensitivity to suxamethonium
U/U	80	60	97%	Normal
A/A	20	20	1:3000	Sensitive, 2h paralysis
A/U	60	50	1:25	Minimal or no prolongation
F/F	65	35	1:150000	Sensitive, 1–2h paralysis
S/S	80	60	Very rare	Sensitive, 3–4h paralysis

H, K and J type have been identified but are rare.
  The present inhibition is usually referred to as the dibucaine number or fluoride number.

Reference

Davis L, Britten J J, Morgan M 1997 Cholinesterase: its significance in anaesthetic practice. Anaesthesia 52: 244–260

RESPIRATORY SYSTEM

ANAESTHESIA – EFFECT ON RESPIRATORY FUNCTION

- FRC reduced
- Change in breathing pattern with predominant diaphragmatic breathing (intercostals more depressed)
- Reduced alveolar ventilation, depressed CO_2 response curve, reduced hypoxic respiratory drive
- Increased shunt (increased (A–a) O_2 difference)
- Increased dead space (physiological dead space)
- Reduced compliance; increased resistance
- Increased $\dot{V}/\dot{Q}$ abnormality (increased (A–a) O_2 difference)
- Cilial paralysis, mucosal drying (anticholinergics, dry gas, nasal bypassing)
- Airway instrumentation and contamination
- Depressed airway reflexes

BRONCHOPLEURAL FISTULA

Usually postoperative (post-pneumonectomy); can also follow abscess formation, neoplasia, bullae or may be traumatic.

Signs

- Postural nocturnal cough
- Copious brown sputum
- Hypoxia and cardiovascular collapse
- Pleural fluid level may be seen to fall
- Methylene blue introduced into the pleural cavity may be expectorated

Management

- Sit patient up with the affected side dependent, also with the fistula clear of pleural fluid if possible (to protect the healthy lung from contamination)
- Increase inspired oxygen fraction (F_iO_2)
- Intravenous access and resuscitation
- Drain pleural cavity

- Early isolation of the fistula (endobronchial intubation)
- Possibly best achieved using a single lumen tube under direct vision

Induction options

- Awake under local anaesthesia (but coughing and contamination still a risk)
- Deep volatile agent (generally unsatisfactory in a shocked patient)
- Rapid sequence (probably the best option in experienced hands)

Restoration of spontaneous ventilation

- Early restoration of spontaneous ventilation or high frequency positive pressure ventilation (HFPPV) to minimize ongoing pressure on the bronchial stump (endobronchial intubation cannot be continued in the long term)

Considerations

- Patients are often elderly
- Poor respiratory reserve (post-pneumonectomy have single lung contaminated following fistula formation. Chronic lung disease is also common in this group of patients, who are usually smokers)
- Tracheal distortion following pneumonectomy (may complicate intubation)
- Patients cannot lie flat for induction
- Pressure (IPPV) on the bronchial stump must be avoided whenever possible

DESIRABLE THEATRE VENTILATOR CHARACTERISTICS

- Reliable, robust, simple
- Control of tidal volume and rate
- Time cycled
- Monitoring of inspiratory pressure and expiratory volume with alarms
- Disconnection, high inspiratory pressure and power failure alarms
- Inspiratory pressure should be limited to avoid barotrauma. Upper limit should be variable to enable asthmatic patients requiring high pressures to be ventilated
- Variable I:E ratio setting
- Able to administer PEEP
- Compatible with humidifiers
- Able to use various gas sources (pipeline and cylinder – 4 bar, air)
- Power source – possible gas powered is best, but dependent on circumstances
- Easily autoclavable gas circuit

- Adaptable for use with a semi-closed circuit
- Adaptable for paediatric use
- Cheap (both to purchase and to maintain)

HYPOCARBIA

Advantages

- Associated hyperventilation ensures good aeration and prevents atelectasis
- Reduces respiratory drive
- May reduce anaesthetic requirement
- Aids hypotension (reduced sympathetic drive, reduced venous return associated with the hyperventilation)
- Reduces CBF and ICP
- Alkalosis (respiratory alkalosis of hypocapnia) is safer than acidosis
- Decreased intraocular pressure

Disadvantages

- Alkalosis shifts the O_2 dissociation curve to the left (increasing Hb affinity and reducing tissue release)
- Decreased venous return and cardiac output may result in reduced blood flow and hypotension
- Excessive intracerebral vasoconstriction (secondary to hypocapnia) may be detrimental
- Hypocapnia results in reduced postoperative respiratory drive with hypoventilation and hypoxia
- Increased risk of seizure when used with higher concentrations of enflurane

HYPOXIA

Subdivisions

- Hypoxic hypoxia (due to low haemoglobin saturation)
- Anaemic hypoxia (due to reduced functioning haemoglobin)
- Stagnant hypoxia (due to failure of sufficient blood to reach tissues)
- Cytotoxic hypoxia (due to inability of tissues to utilize O_2 e.g. cyanide poisoning)

Causes of hypoxic hypoxia

- Reduced alveolar partial pressure of O_2
- Hypoventilation
- $\dot{V}/\dot{Q}$ inequality
- Shunt

- Reduced cardiac output
- Increased tissue requirement

Reduced alveolar partial pressure of O_2
- Resulting from either low pressure, as at altitude, or low percentage of O_2 (such as occurs when there is O_2 supply failure on a Boyle's machine and 100% N_2O is administered), or from dilution of alveolar O_2, e.g. by N_2O in 'diffusion hypoxia'

Hypoventilation
- This occurs according to the alveolar gas equation:

$$P_AO_2 = P_iO_2 - \frac{P_ACO_2}{R}$$

(ignoring the small correction factor (F))
- Important clinical causes of hypoventilation include unrecognized oesophageal intubation, obstructed endotracheal tube or airway, disconnection of ventilator tubing, pneumothorax and central depression

$\dot{V}/\dot{Q}$ inequality
- High $\dot{V}/\dot{Q}$ ratios result when regional perfusion is inadequate to provide blood to take up the O_2 delivered to the alveoli (ventilation is wasted so physiological dead space is increased)
- Low $\dot{V}/\dot{Q}$ ratios result when regional ventilation is inadequate to saturate all the passing blood (perfusion is wasted and unsaturated blood passes the lung so effective shunting occurs)

Shunt
- In pure shunt blood bypasses functioning alveoli, either by flowing through unventilated lung (in contrast to underventilated lung in $\dot{V}/\dot{Q}$ abnormality) or by way of an intracardiac shunt. In contrast to hypoxia due to $\dot{V}/\dot{Q}$ inequality, the hypoxia of shunt is not corrected by breathing 100% O_2

Reduced cardiac output
- If tissue requirements are unchanged where flow is reduced more O_2 will be removed from each 100 ml of perfusing blood so the Po_2 of mixed venous blood will be lower. That venous blood mixing with oxygenated blood (some shunt is always present) will therefore result in a lower P_aO_2 than where the mixed venous blood is more saturated. Obviously this effect is more important when more blood is shunted

Increased tissue requirement
- This occurs, for example, in malignant hyperpyrexia. High tissue uptake will result in a low mixed venous Po_2

Equation to illustrate elements of hypoxia

The elements of hypoxia (except cytotoxic hypoxia) can be appreciated from the oxygen flux equation:

$$\text{tissue oxygen flux} = (\text{Hb}^1 \times 1.34^2 \times \text{saturation}^3) \times \text{blood flow}^4$$

where:

[1] = anaemic hypoxia
[2] = anaemic hypoxia, this is the combining power of haemoglobin in ml O_2/100 ml and when decreased, e.g. by CO, results in a reduction of functioning haemoglobin
[3] = hypoxic hypoxia (causes of reduced haemoglobin saturation as above)
[4] = stagnant hypoxia

Clinical detection of cyanosis

- Observation of patient's colour is generally unsatisfactory (experienced anaesthetists failed to detect cyanosis in 5% of patients with a saturation of 89% or Po_2 7.7 kPa), especially where lighting is poor (e.g. under green towels) and in plethoric patients with peripheral cyanosis. Detection is even more difficult in non-Caucasians

Methods of monitoring

- Pulse oximeter (absorption of light from non-pulsatile tissues is distinguished from that absorbed by arterial blood)
- Blood gas sampling (invasive, intermittent)
- Transcutaneous Po_2 electrode (slow calibration – 20 min, inaccurate with low skin blood flow)
- Direct intra-arterial Po_2 monitoring in neonates using umbilical artery probe
- Disconnection and F_1o_2 alarms (but these do not directly reflect patient's Po_2 levels)

ONE-LUNG ANAESTHESIA

- In the lateral position IPPV will preferentially ventilate the upper lung (since the lower is less compliant with the abdominal contents and mediastinal structures lying on this lung), while blood flow is maximal to the lower lung (determined by gravity). This results in a $\dot{V}/\dot{Q}$ inequality
- Preferential ventilation of the upper lung is further increased once the chest is opened, owing to removal of the negative pleural pressure on that side of the mediastinum (permitting the mediastinum to further compress the dependent lung) and the removal of the chest wall resistance

- Once one-lung anaesthesia is instituted and the lower lung only is ventilated then shunting continues, due to continuing blood flow to the unventilated upper lung. Hypoxia can be severe

Hypoxia of one-lung anaesthesia can be minimized by

Continuation of two-lung anaesthesia
Should be continued for as long as possible.

Increased F_iO_2
It is usual to give 50% O_2 or more.

Restriction or cessation of blood flow to the unventilated upper lung
Early pulmonary artery ligation during pneumonectomy, or retraction of the lung obstructs pulmonary flow where pneumonectomy is not performed.

O_2 insufflation to the unventilated lung
Ensuring that blood passing through this lung will be oxygenated to some extent.

Maintenance of cardiac output
Whenever shunt is present good cardiac output will result in a higher O_2 content of mixed venous blood (less tissue extraction due to more flow), so the resulting reduction of P_aO_2 will be less.

Use of small amount of PEEP
Usually to upper lung but sometimes applied to lower lung with benefit.

Use of left-sided double-lumen tube
To minimize risk of right upper lobe collapse (unless surgery demands use of right-sided tube).

Reference

Conacher I D 2000 Time to apply Occam's razor to failure of hypoxic pulmonary vasoconstriction during one lung ventilation [editorial]. British Journal of Anaesthesia 84(4): 434–436

POSITIONS FOR ANAESTHESIA

Supine

- Decreased FRC (about 30%) on assuming supine position. Further fall on induction of anaesthesia
- Restriction of diaphragmatic movement by abdominal contents (especially in obese patients)

- Trachea angled backward (30°) in supine position so fluids will flow down
- Aortocaval compression (as described in pregnancy) can occur in the obese and in patients with intra-abdominal masses
- Flattening of the lumbar spine with muscle relaxation during anaesthesia, associated with flattening of the lumbar lordosis and postoperative backache

Trendelenburg

- Further decrease of FRC over supine level
- Weight of abdominal contents splints diaphragm; increased work of breathing
- Increased venous return, increased cerebral venous pressure (reduced cerebral perfusion pressure, raised ICP)
- Raised intragastric pressure
- Shoulder pressure can cause brachial plexus injury

Reverse Trendelenburg

- Venous pooling and reduced venous return
- Lesser fall of FRC than in supine position

Lithotomy

- Decreased vital capacity and FRC (restriction of diaphragm, especially in obese patients)
- Increased work of breathing
- Increased intragastric pressure
- Difficulty in turning patients in emergency (legs secured)
- Danger of injuries to hips and backs
- Risk of pressure damage to common peroneal nerve if legs positioned inside poles

Lateral

- Better ventilation in lower lung during spontaneous respiration (lower dome of diaphragm is raised by abdominal contents so greater potential for excursion, also more curved so more force – application of Laplace's Law), also more blood flow to lower lung (gravity effect)
- Lack of stability (patient must be supported)
- Decreased ventilation of lower lung during IPPV leads to increased $\dot{V}/\dot{Q}$ inequality

Prone

- Reduced anteroposterior (AP) chest expansion

- Diaphragmatic excursion can be restricted when support of the shoulders and pelvis is incorrect (especially in obese patients)
- Eyes must be protected from abrasion
- Difficulty in holding on mask and maintaining airway
- Poor access to the endotracheal tube; possibility of tube kinking during positioning
- Brachial plexus damage if arms brought too far forward

Reference

Coonan J J, Hope C E 1983 Cardio-respiratory effects of change of body position. Canadian Anaesthetic Society Journal 30: 4

RIGID BRONCHOSCOPY

- Major indication in fit patients is for removal for foreign body
- Patients requiring bronchoscopy are likely to have impaired respiratory function (collapse/consolidation, bronchopneumonia)
- Patients are frequently smokers with hyperreactive airway reflexes
- There is competition for the airway between the anaesthetist and surgeon
- Bronchospasm and cardiac dysrhythmias are common
- Gas exchange must be maintained (see below)
- Laryngeal reflexes must be abolished for the procedure but should recover rapidly on termination of the bronchoscopy
- The procedure may cause bleeding and bronchial obstruction
- Local anaesthetic toxicity is a risk (4% lidocaine (lignocaine) = 40 mg/ml, metered 10% spray delivers 10 mg per spray: 200 mg is the maximum recommended dose (BNF))
- There is risk of awareness with a general anaesthetic/relaxant technique
- Bronchoscopy can be performed under local anaesthesia or general anaesthesia (the latter is usual for rigid bronchoscopy)
- General anaesthetic techniques include deep anaesthesia with a volatile agent or the use of total intravenous anaesthesia (TIVA)

Methods of ensuring gas exchange in relaxed patients during bronchoscopy

Apnoeic oxygenation
Apnoea with insufflation of O_2 via a catheter to the carina (CO_2 rises at about 0.4 kPa/min during apnoea).

Ventilating bronchoscope
With a glass window on the bronchoscope. Ventilation is not possible when the window is opened, e.g. for biopsy.

Sanders injector

Injection of gas (O_2) at pressure into bronchoscope maintains ventilation (at 410 kPa or 4 bar pressure and a 16 G injection cannula the maximum pressure generated in an unobstructed adult bronchoscope is 30 cmH$_2$O – higher pressures occur if escape of gas from the scope is obstructed).

HFPPV

Results in low airway pressures and does not entrain gas. High flow of gas out of the bronchoscope may be unpleasant for the operator and infected material carried with it may be hazardous (goggles should be worn).

CARDIOVASCULAR SYSTEM

ABDOMINAL AORTIC ANEURYSM

- Patients often elderly, male, hypertensive, diabetic, smokers
- More emergency than elective cases
- Frequent coronary artery disease; often a history of previous myocardial infarction
- Potential large blood loss and massive transfusion
- Preoperative hypertension (associated with tracheal intubation, aortic mobilization and clamping) is undesirable. Postoperative hypertension must be avoided
- Hypotension after declamping should be avoided (avoid acidosis, maintain preload before clamp removed, prefer slow declamping)
- Renal function may be impaired (both preoperatively and as a result of surgery)
- Spinal ischaemia is a risk
- Ileus may be prolonged; the abdominal wound is large; postoperative chest infection is common
- Preoperative shock is also a factor in those who rupture preoperatively
- Temperature must be maintained
- Consider ventilation until temperature and cardiovascular systems stable
- Pain control important, consider epidural for elective cases where no contraindications and for emergency cases postoperatively when stable

Reference

Nimmo A F 2001 Anaesthesia for emergency abdominal aortic aneurysm. Bulletin 5. Royal College of Anaesthesia

COARCTATION OF THE AORTA

- May present with severe cardiac failure in neonates (preductal)

- Bleeding may be profuse from large collateral intercostal vessels (*N.B.* rib notching) as chest is opened and arterial surgery may also be associated with significant blood loss
- Hypertension on aortic clamping may be severe (especially if above subclavian since collaterals occur predominantly via this route)
- Hypotension may occur on unclamping
- Intercostal injections should be avoided
- Hypertension may be a problem postoperatively
- Spinal cord ischaemia is a risk
- There is an association with intracerebral berry aneurysm

CORONARY ARTERY DISEASE

Myocardial ischaemia in cases of coronary artery disease results from an imbalance between oxygen delivery and demand.

O_2 delivery dependent on

- Coronary blood flow = directly related to coronary artery perfusion pressure (CAPP)
- CAPP = aortic diastolic pressure – left ventricular end diastolic pressure (LVEDP)
    = inversely related to the heart rate (shorter diastole with faster rates)
    = inversely related to the coronary vascular resistance (depends on blood viscosity, sympathetic tone and, most importantly, fixed resistance due to atheromatous narrowing)
  N.B. O_2 content = Hb × saturation × capacity
- the optimal level of haematocrit in patients with coronary artery disease is presently unclear. The lower limit of normal haematocrit (30%) is probably a reasonable goal at present, the extent of acceptable variation is unknown

O_2 demand dependent on

- Heart rate
- Systolic BP (afterload)
- Ventricular volume (preload)
- Myocardial contractility

Induction of ischaemia

- Tachycardia and increased LVEDP have greater potential to induce ischaemia (both increase demand and reduce supply) than hypertension (though increasing demand, associated diastolic pressure rise increases CAPP, and so supply). *N.B.* Subendocardium is most vulnerable to ischaemia

Risk factors

Anaesthesia in patients with coronary artery disease
- Unstable angina
- Previous full thickness infarction (Q waves on ECG)
- Diabetes requiring drug therapy
- Heart failure (previous or current), ejection fraction < 35%
- Ventricular dysrhythmia
- Age > 70 years
- Emergency procedure
- Severe aortic stenosis
- Poor general condition
- Intraperitoneal or intrathoracic procedure

Many of these factors are used in the Multifactorial Index of Cardiac Risk suggested by Goldman (1983) (see Core References).

Further factors that may be of importance
- Bundle branch blocks do not appear to increase perioperative risk
- The significance of atrial fibrillation remains unclear (as an independent risk factor)
- Prophylactic glycerol trinitrate (GTN) infusion appears not to effectively reduce the incidence of perioperative ischaemia

Anaesthetic management involves

Maintenance of O_2 supply
- Avoidance of hypoxia, anaemia and hypotension (diastolic). However, obstruction due to atheroma is unrelieved by vasodilators

Reduction of O_2 requirement
- Includes avoidance of tachycardia, hypertension and sympathetic activity (with increased heart rate and systolic BP) and avoidance of undue elevation of the LVEDP (by reduction of preload, e.g. by nitrates). Positive inotropic agents may also decrease O_2 requirement by reducing LVEDP
- Preoperative and perioperative β-adrenoceptor antagonists have clearly been shown to reduce the incidence of perioperative acute myocardial ischaemia in patients with myocardial infarction. Sufficient dosing of opioids prior to induction may also assist to moderate the response to intubation
- It is suggested that heart rate and BP should be maintained within 20% of awake values

Monitoring is important, including
- Pulse

- BP
- Pulse oximetry
- ECG (particularly to detect ischaemia: a V5/CM5 lead detects anterior ischaemia; lead II detects inferior ischaemia)
  N.B.: leads II and III detected only 30% of ischaemic episodes while the addition of V5 detected 75% of electrocardiographically detectable ischaemic events. However, only 20–50% of episodes of ischaemia are associated with any ECG change. New wall motion abnormality detected on echocardiography appears to be a much more sensitive monitor of intra-operative ischaemia
- CVP/pulmonary artery wedge pressure (PAWP) (in selected cases)
  N.B.: while pulmonary artery monitoring may assist with the diagnosis of left ventricular failure or incipient pulmonary oedema, increases in pulmonary arterial wedge pressure has been shown to be an insensitive indicator of myocardial ischaemia in contrast to wall motion abnormality detected by transoesophageal echocardiography
- Rate Pressure Product (RPP) = heart rate × systolic pressure. Monitoring of RPP has been advocated with intervention to maintain value below 12 000

Pharmacological manipulations

Pharmacological manipulations available to treat myocardial ischaemia that is associated with:

↑BP	deepen anaesthesia; vasodilator (arteriolar)
↑HR	deepen anaesthesia; beta-blocker
↑CVP/PAWP	vasodilator (venous); restrict fluid; diuretic; inotropic agent
↓BP	lighten anaesthesia; give fluids (with care and monitoring); inotropic agent or vasopressor

Reference

Warltier D C, Pagel P S, Kerston J R 2000 Approaches to the prevention of perioperative myocardial ischemia. Anesthesiology 92: 253–259

HYPERTENSION

$$BP = CO \times SVR$$

- Potential for both severe hypertension and hypotension during anaesthesia
- Smooth muscle tone increased, possibly with reduced intravascular volume (relaxation results in hypotension)
- Smooth muscle hypertrophy (more constriction and hence greater resistance rises, with marked increase of blood pressure likely, particularly on laryngoscopy and intubation)

- Left ventricular hypertrophy (reduced ventricular compliance, more susceptible to reductions of preload and afterload)
- Increased incidence of atheromatous arterial disease (coronary artery disease, cerebral vascular disease, peripheral vascular disease)
- Increased myocardial oxygen requirement
- Cerebral and renal autoregulation limits set at higher levels
- Hypotensive drug interactions; drug treatment should be continued

Reference

Prys-Roberts C 1984 Anaesthesia and hypertension. British Journal of Anaesthetics
56: 711

HYPOTENSION

Intentional interference with cardiovascular homoeostatic mechanisms to achieve a reduction of blood pressure (BP).

BP = cardiac output (CO) × systemic vascular resistance (SVR)

or, since CO is determined by stroke volume (SV) and heart rate (HR),

$$BP = (SV \times HR) \times SVR.$$

- A reduction of SV, HR or SVR can result in a reduction of BP, but homoeostatic reflexes will usually maintain BP unless attempts are made to influence a number of the factors determining BP
- A combination of pharmacological, physical and postural measures may be simultaneously employed to achieve the desired hypotension
- SVR can be reduced by regional blockage, ganglion blockade, alpha-sympathetic blockade or direct vasodilation (nitroprusside, volatile agent, histamine release)
- SV can be reduced by reduction of venous return or by direct myocardial depression. Venous return can be reduced by venodilation (e.g. by nitroglycerin), a head-up posture, increased intrathoracic pressure (in IPPV). Myocardial depression can be achieved by beta-blockade or by the use of higher concentrations of volatile agents
- HR can be decreased by beta-blockade or regional sympathetic block above the T4 level
- Elevation of the operative site above the heart will further decrease arterial pressure at the site and will reduce venous pressure and subsequent oozing
- Hypoxia occurs in hypotension, possibly due to inhibition of hypoxic pulmonary vasoconstriction and increased shunting through the lungs
- Drug-induced hypotension is better tolerated than the haemorrhagic type. In normotensive young patients autoregulation is maintained when the mean BP is > 60 mmHg, accordingly a mean pressure of

50 mmHg appears to be a reasonably safe lower limit (also supported by direct assessment of tissue hypoxia)
- Intracranial pressure is abolished while the dura is opened and so mean arterial pressure = cerebral perfusion pressure (normally cerebral perfusion pressure = mean arterial pressure – intracranial pressure); thus lower levels of BP may be tolerated while the dura is opened
- In hypertensive patients autoregulation of cerebral flow operates at higher BP levels. Thus autoregulation may fail with resulting low flow and ischaemia at levels of BP which would be tolerated by non-hypertensive subjects
- When hypotension is employed it is important to monitor patients closely. Since arterial pressure at the level of the brain is most frequently of greatest concern it is suggested that the transducer used to monitor pressure should be sited at the level of the brain (rather than the level of the heart)

MITRAL STENOSIS

Generally due to rheumatic heart disease. Since rheumatic fever is now rare in the UK and symptoms usually take about 20 years to develop, patients tend to be elderly.

Clinical features

- Dyspnoea on exertion (often first noticeable when patients go into atrial fibrillation)
- Atrial fibrillation
- Systemic embolus (from clot which occurs in the distended atrium when it ceases to contract regularly with the onset of fibrillation)
- Haemoptysis (due to raised pulmonary venous pressure and pulmonary hypertension in later stages)
- Patients with significant mitral stenosis are usually treated with a combination of diuretic, digoxin and oral anticoagulant

Clinical signs

- Small volume arterial pulse
- Opening snap in early diastole (unless the valve is calcified)
- Rumbling diastolic murmur (with presystolic accentuation when in sinus rhythm – due to acceleration of flow with atrial contraction)

Effects

- Stenosis of the mitral valve results in an increased left atrial pressure. This, in turn, results in pulmonary oedema and, when chronic, in pulmonary arterial hypertension
- Pulmonary congestion results in reduced compliance

Anaesthetic considerations

- The valvular obstruction results in a fixed CO; thus SVR must be maintained since CO cannot increase to compensate and maintain the BP (BP = CO × SVR)
- Ventricular filling across the obstructed valve depends on a high atrial pressure; the preload must therefore be maintained (symptoms are often precipitated or worsened by the onset of atrial fibrillation)
- Control of the heart rate must be maintained. A rapid heart rate results in a reduced diastolic time for ventricular filling and reduced CO
- Hypoxia must be avoided. The cardiac output is low, resulting in a lower mixed venous Po_2 (and so greater reduction of the P_aO_2 resulting from shunting) and also greater liability to tissue hypoxia due to reduced flow. The pulmonary vascular bed is hypertrophied in cases of pulmonary hypertension and pulmonary vascular resistance may become grossly elevated when patients become hypoxic (or acidotic)

MITRAL REGURGITATION

May be rheumatic (when mitral stenosis is usually associated). Other causes include papillary muscle dysfunction, bacterial endocarditis and dilation of the valve ring in heart failure.

Clinical features

- Dyspnoea
- Fatigue
- Palpitations

Clinical signs

- Left ventricular dilatation and hypertrophy
- Systolic murmur (classically pansystolic) at the apex, radiating to the axilla

Effects

- There is reduced left ventricular stroke volume delivered to the aorta with left atrial fluid overload
- In chronic cases dilation of the atrium limits pressure rise. But in acute cases pulmonary capillary pressure rise is marked with associated severe pulmonary oedema
- Large V waves are seen on PAWP trace
- The ventricular overload is volume not pressure so ischaemia is not a prominent feature (though the LVEDP is high, reducing blood flow,

myocardial oxygen consumption is more influenced by pressure work)

Anaesthetic considerations

- The fraction of blood regurgitating depends on:
  — The size of the mitral valve orifice during systole
  — The heart rate (slow rates are associated with more regurgitation)
  — The pressure gradient across the valve
  — The relative resistances of flow to the aorta and atrium (a low SVR favours forward flow to the aorta)
- During anaesthesia mild increases of heart rate and falls of SVR are desirable
- Excessive myocardial depression should be avoided; however, low concentrations of volatile agent are generally well tolerated
- Antibiotic prophylaxis for bacterial endocarditis is indicated

AORTIC STENOSIS

Often due to calcification of the abnormal (usually bicuspid) aortic valve. Rheumatic aortic stenosis is almost invariably associated with mitral valve disease.

Clinical features

- Classical symptoms include angina, dyspnoea on exertion and syncope (characteristically on effort), but these are late features
- Sudden death

Clinical signs

- Pulse is characteristically low-volume and slow-rising
- Small pulse pressure
- Left ventricular hypertrophy
- Crescendo–decrescendo systolic murmur, loudest over the second right intercostal space radiating to neck with a thrill over the same area

Effects

- Reduction of the normal $3 \, cm^2$ aortic valve area by 25% usually results in symptoms
- A systolic gradient of 50 mmHg or more across the valve is considered significant stenosis
- Angina results from increased O_2 demand (increased muscle mass, increased ventricular wall tension) with reduced supply (reduced diastolic pressure, raised LVEDP)

Anaesthetic considerations

- Thick ventricle is of reduced compliance so atrial contraction is important for optimal ventricular filling (so patients must be maintained in sinus rhythm) and preload must be maintained
- The reduced ventricular compliance requires a higher PAWP to maintain CO
- Tachycardia must be avoided (less time to eject blood through stenosis, less time for ventricular filling during shorter diastole, increased likelihood of myocardial ischaemia)
- Fixed CO so SVR must not be acutely reduced since CO cannot be increased to maintain BP (BP = CO × SVR) and gross hypotension will ensue. At the same time a high afterload (SVR) opposes forward flow across the valve and increases ventricular pressure which can precipitate myocardial ischaemia
- Aortic diastolic pressure must be maintained to preserve coronary artery blood flow
- Myocardial depression should be avoided
- Antibiotic prophylaxis for bacterial endocarditis is indicated
- Postoperatively, patients often require antihypertensive therapy

AORTIC REGURGITATION

Acute causes include dissection of the thoracic aorta and bacterial endocarditis. Chronic cases include rheumatic heart disease (when mitral valve disease is usually associated), hypertension, syphilis.

Clinical features

- Classically few until dyspnoea develops

Clinical signs

- Collapsing pulse ('water hammer')
- Wide pulse pressure, cardiac dilatation
- Early diasystolic murmur at the lowest left sternum (best heard during expiration)
- Left ventricular hypertrophy

Effects

- Magnitude of regurgitation depends on:
  — Heart rate (long diastole in bradycardia gives longer for regurgitation to occur)
  — The diastolic aortic pressure
  — The size of the orifice during diastole

- The volume overload of the ventricle results in hypertrophy in chronic cases but ischaemia is not a prominent finding (pressure work is low). However, the aortic diastolic pressure is low and LVEDP is high so myocardial flow may be impaired

Anaesthetic considerations

- Slight tachycardia is desirable
- Reduction of the SVR can improve forward flow
- Antibiotic prophylaxis for bacterial endocarditis is indicated

LEFT-TO-RIGHT SHUNT

- Causes include atrioseptal defect (ASD), ventricular septal defect (VSD), patent ductus arteriosus (PDA)
- Results in increased pulmonary blood flow and decreased systemic flow
- The degree of shunting depends on:
  — The size of the orifice
  — The relative pressures on each side
  — The relative resistances on each side

Anaesthetic considerations

- Reduced SVR and increased PVR reduces the shunt and is desirable (IPPV increases PVR, surgical banding of the pulmonary artery has the same effect)
- Antibiotic prophylaxis for bacterial endocarditis is indicated

RIGHT-TO-LEFT SHUNT

- Causes include Fallot's tetralogy, Eisenmenger's syndrome (reversal of a L–R shunt due to an irreversible increase of pulmonary pressure), Ebstein's abnormality of the tricuspid valve
- Results in decreased pulmonary blood flow and diversion of unsaturated blood to the systemic circulation (with cyanosis)
- The degree of shunting depends on:
  — The size of the orifice
  — The relative pressures on each side
  — The relative resistances on each side

Anaesthetic considerations

- Increased SVR and decreased PVR reduces the shunt and is desirable (IPPV increases PVR so inflation pressures should be low). The squatting posture characteristic of children with Fallot's tetralogy is thought to compress the femoral arteries and to increase SVR

- Flow from the right to left can deliver air which has been injected into the systemic circulation (small bubbles usually filtered by the lung with no demonstrable detrimental effect). Great care must be exercised in cases of R–L shunt
- Antibiotic prophylaxis for bacterial endocarditis is indicated

CARDIAC TAMPONADE

Causes include trauma, pericarditis, uraemia.

Clinical features and signs

- Tachycardia
- Pulsus paradoxus
- Kussmaul's sign

Effects

- Tachycardia, vasoconstriction and increased venous return in attempt to maintain BP
- Pulse volume decreases on inspiration, probably because the descending diaphragm increases the intrapericardiac pressure and reduces ventricular filling (pulsus paradoxus)
- CVP increases on inspiration for same reason

Anaesthetic considerations

- Maintain tachycardia
- Maintain SVR. Fixed CO so SVR must not be acutely reduced since CO cannot be increased to maintain BP (BP = CO × SVR) and gross hypotension will ensue
- Small tidal volumes to minimize effect of respiratory induced impairment of venous return and ventricular filling
- Consider drainage of tamponade, where appropriate, before induction

HAEMATOLOGY

ANAEMIA

Effects

Reduction of the number of circulating erythrocytes resulting in a reduced haemoglobin concentration and consequently reduced O_2 carrying capacity. Reduced O_2 carrying capacity will result in reduced O_2 delivery to the tissues unless flow is increased, as illustrated by the O_2 flux equation:

$$O_2 \text{ flux} = Hb \times \text{saturation} \times 1.34^1 \times \text{cardiac output}$$

$$(+ \text{ dissolved } O_2 \text{ in solution}^2)$$

where:

^{1} = amount of O_2 (ml) carried per g haemoglobin and
^{2} = 0.3 ml/100 ml/13.3 kPa of O_2 tension.

The normal O_2 content is 20 ml/100 ml and 5 ml/100 ml is normally extracted (i.e. this is the normal arteriovenous difference). There is, therefore, a significant margin of safety before normal patients develop tissue hypoxia in situations of anaemia.

Changes in chronic anaemia which improve tissue oxygenation
- Shift of the O_2 dissociation curve to the right (due to increased 2,3-DPG)
- Increased cardiac output (significant when Hb < 9 g/100 ml)
- Reduced viscosity improves flow (O_2 delivery optimal at 11 g/100 ml, haematocrit 30%)
- Renal erythropoietin production stimulates erythropoiesis

Principles of management
- Transfusion where severe (at least 24 h preoperatively to permit fluid equilibration and restoration of 2,3-DPG levels in transfused cells)
- Hypoxia must be avoided; preoxygenation should be performed before induction of anaesthesia
- Increased F_iO_2
- Smoking should be avoided (carboxyhaemoglobin may constitute up to 15% of haemoglobin in smokers)
- Cardiac output must be maintained
- Shifts of the O_2 dissociation curve to the left must be avoided as this decreases release of O_2 to tissues (left shift results from hypocapnia, reduced temperature and alkalosis)
- Blood loss must be replaced promptly
- Shivering and increased temperature must be avoided as this markedly increases tissue O_2 consumption
- In cases of megaloblastic anaemia due to vitamin B_{12} deficiency, neuropathy can occur making regional anaesthesia unwise. N_2O has been shown to oxidize vitamin B_{12}, inhibiting methionine synthetase and resulting in megaloblastic anaemia in chronically exposed patients. Avoidance of N_2O may thus be wise in cases of vitamin B_{12} deficiency

MASSIVE BLOOD TRANSFUSION

- Defined as:
  — Replacement of patient blood volume in 24 h
  — Transfusion where half blood volume replaced during surgery

- Good venous access is needed to enable adequate volume to be administered to compensate for loss. Spasm of peripheral veins (in response to cold blood and shock) may limit flow; access to central veins is advisable, as is the use of more than one large cannula in situ:
  — Remember flow directly related to length of tube, viscosity of fluid, pressure gradient and inversely proportional to the fourth power of the radius (Poiseuille), hence radius most important
- Pressure infusion equipment and blood warmers should be available
- Monitoring is important, both to evaluate the effects of blood loss and transfusion and to protect the patient during anaesthesia while the anaesthetist is occupied with replacing blood loss (such events as disconnection are more likely to be overlooked):
  — Blood pressure – arterial monitoring indicated
  — ECG
  — Pulse oximetry
  — Full gas monitoring including $ETCO_2$
  — CVP
  — Urinary output
  — Temperature
  — Amount and type of fluid given
  — Consider oesophageal Doppler probe or pulmonary artery catheter
  N.B. Beware blood spillage, sharps and wear gloves

Complications

Cold
Blood is stored at 4°C and administration of large volumes cools the patient. Cold shifts the oxyhaemoglobin dissociation curve to the left. Blood warming units should be employed (but can increase resistance and reduce the rate at which blood can be given).

Citrate
Blood preservatives contain citrate as an anticoagulant. This is normally metabolized rapidly to bicarbonate in the liver. In liver failure, renal failure and hypothermia such metabolism may not occur, leading to citrate toxicity (acidosis and binding of serum calcium).

Acidosis
Blood has a pH of <7.0 at 14 days of storage, due to anaerobic cell metabolism with lactate production. In practice acidosis is unusual in patients after transfusion.

Clotting factors
Factors VIII and V reduce on storage. About 20% of these are present at 21 days in citrate phosphate dextrose (CPD) blood. The amounts present in saline adenine glucose mannitol (SAGM) blood are considerably less. These

factors are present in fresh frozen plasma (FFP) which should be administered to patients receiving large transfusions.

Clotting factors have a wide normal range (V and VIII can fall to 20% without problems in presence of normal haematocrit and platelet count).

Giving FFP was at the rate of 4:1 (4 whole blood to 1 FFP), complicated now with plasma reduced blood; perhaps should be 5:2 once one blood volume has been replaced and there is no prospect of bringing bleeding under control.

Platelets
Functional platelets are absent from blood stored for > 24 h at 4°C. Blood transfusion will thus result in a dilutional thrombocytopenia; however, there are reserves and a platelet count of 40% of initial values is possible where the total circulating blood volume has been transfused.

Platelet function is inversely related to the haematocrit and is compounded by thrombocytopenia below 100×10^9 per litre which results in a progressively prolonged bleeding time. In injury (especially head injury) we should therefore endeavour to keep haematocrit above 30 and platelets above 100.

Platelet counts of 100 can be anticipated when 1–1.5 blood volumes have been transfused. Haematologists say indication for transfusion is a count of 50 accompanied by abnormal bleeding.

Reduced 2,3-DPG levels
Stored red cells have a low 2,3-DPG content (not significantly so for more than 2 weeks in the case of blood stored in CPD but within 1 week in SAGM), which results in a shift to the left of the oxyhaemoglobin dissociation curve and consequently a reduced P_{50} value.

Calcium
Infusion of citrate-containing blood was thought to result in hypocalcaemia; however, mobilization of calcium ion from skeletal stores appears to be rapid and hypocalcaemia is not a problem.

Potassium
Stored blood has a high potassium content (about 30 mmol/l by 21 days of storage); however, hyperkalaemia is unusual, possibly because both warming and increased metabolic activity of the red cells result in reuptake of potassium into these cells.

Risk of reaction
Reactions are more likely where multiple units of blood are transfused, as is the risk of administering the wrong blood (crossmatched for a different patient). Reactions can be classified as:

• Allergic (reaction to plasma protein or leucocyte antigens)
• Febrile (non-specific fever)

- Haemolytic due to mismatch (back pain, renal failure and disseminated intravascular coagulation are other features)

All blood transfused must be checked by two people and carefully documented.

Sensitization
Transfusion of large volumes of blood, especially uncrossmatched group O blood, may result in antibody formation and subsequent difficulties with crossmatching problems. Rhesus-negative women may have to be given Rhesus-positive blood in an emergency when Rhesus-negative blood is unavailable in adequate quantity; sensitization will occur.

Risk of air embolus
Rapid infusion of fluids from multiple drips under pressure makes accidental air embolus more likely. Also, disconnection of a central venous line in a patient with low central venous pressure may permit aspiration of air to the venous system.

Infection
Viral hepatitis, cytomegalovirus (CMV) and Epstein–Barr virus (EBV) may be transmitted. Blood is screened for hepatitis B, hepatitis C, syphilis and HIV. Danger of new variant CJD has led to requirement that the unit number of each bag of blood given is fully documented and kept for at least 11 years in the patient's notes.

Microaggregates
Stored blood contains aggregates of > 200 μm, which it is clearly of benefit to remove. No blood should be given through a giving set which does not include a 170 μm filter. Filtration of smaller aggregates is more controversial; screen and depth filters which remove small (down to 40 μm) aggregates are available but with the advent of SAGM blood are no longer necessary.

Also note Serious Hazards of Transfusion (SHOT Reports 1996–8)
- 366 reports received, 22 deaths
- 52% of patients received blood component intended for someone else
- Collection of blood from its storage site is a major source of primary error
- One fatal case was due to bedside transposition of samples taken for crossmatch, therefore awareness of ABO incompatibility important
- Blood transfusion, while extremely safe, has several potentially fatal hazards
- All staff handling blood should be aware of the importance of correct identity of sample, patient, and blood bag at all stages
- Resources should be directed to evaluation of methods for improving identification of patients

- Acute fever or collapse during or after transfusion may be due to ABO incompatibility or bacterial contamination
- Microbiological complications of transfusion accounted for a minor component of all reports

Reference

Donaldson M D J, Seaman M J, Park G R 1992 Massive blood transfusion. British Journal of Anaesthesia 69: 621–630

PORPHYRIA

- Mostly autosomal dominant inheritance with variable expression
- Classified into acute and non-acute; acute forms problem for anaesthesia
- Porphyrins are essential for formation of haemoglobin, myoglobin and cytochromes
- Glycine + succinyl CoA conversion to aminolaevulinic acid occurs in the liver and bone marrow and is catalysed by delta aminolaevulinic acid synthetase (delta-ALA synthetase); this pathway then continues with the production of porphyrins
- Several types of porphyria are recognized; acute intermittent porphyria is commonest in the UK, produces severest symptoms and can be fatal
- Probably due to decrease in activity of porphobilinogen deaminase
- Characterized by intermittent excretion of porphyrins in the urine or faeces

Acute episodes precipitated by

- Barbiturates
- Etomidate
- Sulphonamides
- Verapamil
- Nifedipine
- Diltiazem
- Aminophylline
- Contraceptive pill
- Pregnancy
- Steroids
- Infection
- Starvation and dehydration – avoid lengthy preoperative starvation

Clinical features

- Abdominal pain and vomiting
- Peripheral neuropathy with weakness or paralysis. May affect autonomic nervous system and cranial nerves

- Confusion or psychosis
- Tachycardia and hypertension
- Dehydration and electrolyte disturbance

During attacks

Increase in urinary porphobilinogen (PBG) and delta aminolaevulinic acid (ALA), also increase in faecal porphyrins.

Detection

- PBG – darkens urine on standing, detected by Ehrlich's aldehyde reagent
- Porphyrins – fluoresce in ultraviolet (UV) light
- Diagnosis is made biochemically by demonstrating low levels of porphobilinogen activity in the erythrocytes

Safe drugs

- Opiates – morphine, fentanyl, codeine
- Propofol
- N_2O
- Volatile agents
- Depolarizing and non-depolarizing muscle relaxants
- Anticholinergics
- Anticholinesterases
- Midazolam
- Salbutamol
- Ranitidine
- Local anaesthetics – lidocaine (lignocaine), bupivacaine

Reference

James M F M, Hift R J 2000 Porphyrias. British Journal of Anaesthesia 85: 143–153

SICKLE CELL ANAEMIA

Hereditary anaemia prevalent in West Africa, the West Indies, Greece, India and among Americans of African origin.

- Results from a defect in the beta-globulin chain of haemoglobin with a single amino acid substitution of valine for glutamic acid. This substitution results in polar cross-linking between haemoglobin chains and tactoid (crystal) formation (sickling) under conditions of hypoxia (i.e. deoxygenated haemoglobin)
- Tactoid formation causes an increase in viscosity and cell fragility
- HbSS (homozygote) sickles at Po_2 of 5 kPa (95% HbS, 5% HbF)

- HbSA (heterozygote) sickles at Po_2 of 2.5 kPa (20–50% HbS)

Sickling tendency depends on

- Percentage of HbS present (95% in homozygous, 25–45% in heterozygous)
- pH
- Presence of other haemoglobins (HbF protects against sickling, HbC makes sickling more likely than when HbA is present)

Clinical features

Heterozygous
- Asymptomatic, no abnormal signs

Homozygous
- Anaemia, fever pains, jaundice
- Skull bossing ('hair on end' appearance on X-ray)
- Overgrowth of the maxilla
- Infarcts (especially spleen and kidney)
- Osteomyelitis
- Leg ulcers
- Gallstones (bilirubin secondary to haemolysis)

Investigations

- Haemoglobin
- Blood film (Hb > 10 g/100 ml and normal film makes homozygous anaemia unlikely)
- Sickle preparation (Sickledex = saponin to lyse cells and hypochlorite-reducing agent to provoke in vitro sickling)
- Haemoglobin electrophoresis

Prevention of sickling

Avoid:

- Hypoxia
- Acidosis
- Stasis (reduced cardiac output, tourniquet)
- Increased viscosity (dehydration, cold)

Management

- Avoid general anaesthesia where possible
- Increased F_iO_2 (including postoperatively)
- Liberal fluids

- Warming
- Maintain cardiac output
- No tourniquet
- Consider alkalinization (shifts O_2 dissociation curve to left, keeps haemoglobin oxygenated at expense of tissues)
- Consider transfusion:
  — Reduces HbS percentage
  — Low 2,3-DPG in stored blood increases O_2 affinity
  — Reduces marrow output of abnormal Hb

However, stored blood is acidotic and cold; transfusion also increases viscosity. Usually reserved for patients with an Hb of < 8 g/100 ml

Reference

Searle J F 1973 Anaesthesia in sickle cell states. Anaesthesia 28: 48–58

STORED BLOOD AND BLOOD PRODUCTS

- 450 ml collected from each donation into 63 ml of preservative
- Fresh blood can be stored for 24 h
- Preservative mixture of citrate-phosphate-dextrose plus adenine – CPDa
- Shelf life 5 weeks (75% viable red cells)
- Lower haematocrit (35–42%) due to dilution by preservative
- Each unit contains about 200 ml of red cells ≈200 mg iron
- Stored at 4°C ± 2°C controlled environment:
  — No ice box
  — Fan circulation of cool air
  — Temperature gauge and pen recorder
  — Alarm for drift of temperature
- Tested for syphilis, Hep B, Hep C, CMV, HIV

Red cell concentrate (packed cells)

- 150–200 ml of plasma removed from whole blood
- Haematocrit about 70%

Saline-adenine-glucose-mannitol (SAG-M) – now main blood type supplied

- Red cells resuspended to a haematocrit of >> 60%
- Increases yield of plasma
- Good red cell survival after 35 days storage
- Viscosity comparable to that of whole blood
- Poor 2,3-DPG survival
- Reduced clotting factors

Fresh frozen plasma

- Prepared within 6 h of donation
- Contains 80–90% of all clotting factors
- Thawed prior to delivery to ward

Cryoprecipitate

- Prepared by carefully thawing fresh frozen plasma and keeping temperature < 4°C
- Sludge forms that can be centifuged out to give about 30 ml of cryoprecipitate
- Contains factor VIII, fibrinogen and cold-insoluble globulin
- Stored at –30°C for up to 6 months

Platelet concentrates

- Old system 6×10^{10} platelets in 50 ml, stored at 22°C, shelf life 3–5 days
- Now issued in adult therapeutic doses (ATD) – 200 ml pack containing the platelets of four donors (unless prepared by single donor apheresis – about 30%)
- In vivo activity is estimated to be 75–80% so one ATD has activity of three units of donated blood

Plasma protein fraction

- Obtain from platelet-poor plasma
- Pasteurized (heated to 60°C for 10 h)

INTENSIVE CARE

BURNS

Mortality

- Mortality related to age of patient and area of burn
- Tables available to predict outcome in relation to these factors
- Latest research suggests further relationship with carboxyhaemoglobin level on admission

Initial treatment

- Resuscitation – Airway, Breathing and Circulation
- Assessment of depth and area of burn (Rule of Nines)

- Assess involvement of respiratory tract – presence of carbon in mouth and nares (indication for early intubation)
- Pain relief
- Catheterize to monitor urine output
- Nasogastric tube to prevent acute dilatation of stomach
- Commence prophylactic treatment to prevent stress ulcers

Fluid replacement

- Controversy over use of colloid or crystalloid (published results show equal success of both techniques; colloid favoured in UK)
- Monitor replacement by:
  — Haematocrit
  — Electrolytes
  — Urine output
  — Pulse and BP
  — CVP
- Adjust fluid accordingly

Nutrition

- Increased requirement for N_2 and calories
- As soon as gastric motility returns, oral diet should be commenced, until then parenteral nutrition will be required

Temperature control

- Danger of heat loss: nurse in warm environment (will also decrease metabolic rate)

Anaesthetic considerations

- Analgesia or anaesthesia may be required for burn dressings
- Use of inhalation techniques: Entonox, enflurane and isoflurane
- Use of IV agents such as ketamine
- Definitive surgery:
  — Difficulty with site of burn and donor areas
  — Venous access
  — Monitoring access
  — Central lines – infection risk
  — Potential for large blood loss
  — Heat loss
  — Intubation difficulty
- Avoid use of suxamethonium because of problem of hyperkalaemia between 48h and about 6 months from the time of the injury

Reference

MacLennan N, Heimbach D M, Cullen B F 1998 Anesthesia for major thermal injury. Anesthesiology 89: 749–770

CRITERIA FOR BRAIN DEATH

Preconditions to be met before testing

- Deep coma and apnoeic
- Irremediable structural damage to the brain
- Reversible causes of brain-stem depression have been excluded:
  — Hypothermia
  — Gross metabolic imbalance
  — Depressant drugs
  — Muscle relaxants

Tests

There must be no response to any of these (note spinal reflexes are permissible).

Reflex responses
- Pupils to light
- Corneal reflex
- Gag reflex
- Facial muscles in response to pain (response within cranial nerve distribution)
- Caloric vestibulo-ocular reflex. Visualize tympanic membrane then syringe 20 ml of ice-cold water into auditory meatus and observe for eye movement

Respiration
- Must prove patient to be apnoeic
- Aim is to disconnect patient from ventilator and allow $P_a\text{CO}_2$ to increase to > 8 kPa
- Disconnect and supply O_2 at 6 l/min via a tracheal catheter and observe patient for 10 min. Monitor saturation by pulse oximetry throughout and check arterial blood gas at conclusion of test
- Special consideration is required for patients with chronic respiratory insufficiency

Repetition of tests
- Tests should be performed on two occasions by two doctors of adequate experience
- They should not be associated with transplant team if organs are for donation

DESIRABLE INTENSIVE CARE VENTILATOR CHARACTERISTICS

Modes

A ventilator for intensive care is generally expected to be able to operate in the following modes:

Controlled mechanical ventilation
Volume preset, flow generation. No facility for spontaneous ventilation.

Triggering (otherwise called assist-control)
Initiation of inhalation by the patient triggers a breath of preset volume.

Intermittent mandatory volume (IMV)
Permits the patient to breathe spontaneously between preset (mandatory) mechanical breaths. To avoid mechanical breaths falling at the peak of a spontaneous inhalation, or in opposition to spontaneous exhalation, the mechanical breaths can be synchronized to coincide with the initiation of a spontaneous breath (SIMV).

Pressure support
The patient initiates inspiration and the ventilator delivers gas flow to maintain a preset positive airway pressure.

Pressure control
The ventilator delivers gas flow to maintain a preset positive airway pressure at a regular preset rate irrespective of patient inspiratory effort.

Desirable Characteristics

- Reliable, robust, simple
- Control of tidal volume, rate, inspiratory flow and pattern
- Adjustable I:E ratio
- Time cycled
- PEEP and CPAP facility
- Minimal additional work of breathing in spontaneous breathing modes (SIMV, CPAP)
  — Features such as continuous flow and flow triggering are associated with a reduced work of breathing
- A facility to set an end-inspiratory plateau (or hold). An inspiratory plateau may improve ventilation of alveoli with long time constants and reduce shunt. Mean intrathoracic pressure is increased and venous return may be reduced
- An ability reliably to deliver a range of oxygen concentrations from 21% to 100%

- A facility to increase oxygen to 100% for a preset period to cover suctioning, and then to revert to the previous concentration
- Inspiratory pressure should be capable of limitation to avoid barotrauma. Upper limit should be variable to enable asthmatic patients requiring high pressures to be ventilated
- Monitoring of inspiratory pressure and expiratory volume with alarms
- Compatibility with humidifiers and integral nebulization (i.e. the nebulizer is run from the set tidal volume at the set oxygen percentage)
- Gas circuit should be easily sterilized to avoid cross-infection
- Adaptable for paediatric use
- A sigh function is commonly incorporated. Sighs are programmed periodic hyperinflations which are intended to prevent progressive atelectasis. Sighs are poorly tolerated by patients and where large tidal volumes are used and regular physiotherapy is given, sighs are probably not necessary and are now infrequently used
- An ability to display monitored information graphically
- An ability to calculate and display derived respiratory measurements (resistance, compliance, auto-PEEP, oxygen consumption, etc.)
- Disconnection and power failure alarms
- Cheap (both to purchase and to maintain)

MANAGEMENT OF DIABETIC KETOACIDOSIS

Fundamental principles

- Replace fluid loss
- Replace electrolyte loss
- Restore normal carbohydrate metabolism
- Treat underlying cause

Fluid

Normal saline or $1/2$ normal saline if significant hyperosmolality (> 320 mosmol/kg).

Potassium

Total body potassium depleted due to osmotic diuresis but plasma levels are increased as a consequence of acidosis. Early replacement is required and levels monitored regularly (at least 1–2-hourly during the acute stage).

Phosphate, magnesium

Both phosphate and magnesium are lost with osmotic diuresis. Phosphate falls further as hyperglycaemia and fluid depletion are corrected.

Insulin infusion

Adjusted according to response. 5IU/h is a reasonable starting rate (intramuscular insulin is less reliable in shocked patients and is not now commonly used).

Bicarbonate

Controversial and potentially dangerous. Has not been shown to enhance ketone clearance or rate of recovery.

Glucose

Glucose should be administered when the blood glucose level falls to 15mmol/l or less. The insulin infusion should be continued since glucose falls more rapidly than ketones.

Monitoring

- Intravascular volume replacement assessment:
  — HR
  — BP
  — Hourly urine
  — CVP
- ABG (hourly)
- Blood sugar (hourly)
- Potassium (hourly, then 2–4-hourly)
- Sodium, creatinine (on admission and repeated if abnormal)
- Phosphate (every 4–8h)
- FBC and film* (on admission)
- Blood and other cultures as clinically indicated
- ECG (12-lead and continuous)
- CXR

MANAGEMENT OF ACUTE SEVERE ASTHMA

Oxygen

- Hypoxia is common since $\dot{V}/\dot{Q}$ mismatch is marked. Additional oxygen is indicated

Nebulized beta$_2$-agonist agents (e.g. salbutamol)

- Standard therapy

---

* Neutrophilia is a common association of ketoacidosis in the absence of infection but toxic changes and left shift suggest infection.

- Note that nebulized particles which are not at body temperature or iso-osmolar have been shown to exacerbate bronchospasm

Ipratropium bromide

- Anticholinergic without systemic effect and which does not inhibit mucociliary clearance
- Some synergistic bronchodilation with salbutamol

Corticosteroids

- Of increased importance now that the inflammatory features of severe asthma are recognized
- Optimal dose or agent not established

Aminophylline

- Synergism with beta-agonist drugs is debatable and its role in acute asthma is questioned; if used, levels should be monitored

Intravenous beta$_2$-agonist agents (e.g. salbutamol)

- When severity of bronchospasm prevents effective delivery of nebulized drug to the distal airways
- Lactic acidosis is a recognized complication of high-dose salbutamol therapy

Adrenaline (epinephrine)

- May be indicated in extreme cases, particularly those with extremely rapid onset

Ketamine

- Sympathomimetic action has led to suggestions that this is the optimal induction agent and/or sedation in ventilated asthmatics

Antihistamines

- Not shown to be effective

Mechanical ventilation

- Should be adjusted to avoid gas trapping as this has been shown to correlate with the development of barotrauma (including pneumothorax) and hypotension

- Ventilator settings which optimize expiratory time result in least gas trapping
- Monitoring of the trapped volume is advocated

References

Jain S, Hanania N A, Guntupalli K K 1998 Ventilation of patients with asthma and obstructive lung disease. Critical Care Clinics 14(4): 685–705

Lipworth B J 1997 Treatment of acute asthma. Lancet 350(11): 1823

PHOSPHATE

- Average body phosphorus = 712 g (28 000 mmol)
- Distribution:
  - 85% stored in bone as hydroxyapatite crystals
  - 14% stored in soft tissues as phosphate
  - 1% in the blood
- Soft tissue phosphate
  - Factor in intermediate metabolism
  - Component in genetic material
- Structural component (phospholipids)
  - Most abundant intracellular anion (100 mmol/l) (i.e. 100 × plasma concentration)
  - Only small fraction of intracellular phosphate is in the inorganic form – majority in intermediary carbohydrates, lipids and proteins
- Phosphate in blood exists in both organic (2/3) and inorganic (1/3) forms with a total plasma concentration of 3.9 mmol/l (laboratories normally measure inorganic form)
- Intake 800–1200 g/day
- Homeostasis controlled by parathyroid hormone 1,25-dihydroxycholecalciferol and calcitonin and involves intestine, kidneys and bone
- Uptake throughout bowel but mainly jejunum by sodium dependant active transport in proximal bowel and passive diffusion of phosphate ions in jejunum and ileum
- Physiological functions
  - Source of high-energy bonds of adenosine triphosphate (ATP)
  - Vital component of many intracellular compounds – phospholipids, nucleic acids, etc.
  - Important role as intracellular messenger – cyclic adenosine monophosphate
  - Component of 2,3-DPG
  - Regulator of enzymes in the glycolytic pathway
  - Acts as buffer for plasma pH
  - Role in many functions of the immune system

PULMONARY ARTERY CATHETERIZATION

Various information can be derived from a pulmonary artery catheter (Swan–Ganz):

- Pulmonary artery pressures (systolic and diastolic)
- Pulmonary artery wedge pressure
- Cardiac output
- Mixed venous oxygen saturation

Pulmonary artery pressures

- Identifies the presence or development of pulmonary hypertension
- In the absence of increased pulmonary resistance the pulmonary artery end diastolic pressure (PAEDP) is about 1–3 mmHg higher than the PAWP (N.B. the PAWP can never be higher than the PAEDP)
- Poor correlation between the CVP and PAWP have been demonstrated in critically ill patients. In this situation PAWP is preferred for assessment of fluid management

Pulmonary artery wedge pressure (PAWP)

- PAWP gives an indirect measurement of the left atrial pressure (LAP) which equates to the left ventricular end diastolic pressure (LVEDP)
- High ventilation pressures, increased pulmonary vascular resistance and mitral stenosis cause the LVEDP to be lower than the measured PAWP

Cardiac output

- Incorporation of a thermistor at the tip of the pulmonary artery catheter permits measurement of cardiac output using the thermodilution technique
- A volume of cold saline is injected into the right atrium and the temperature drop at the thermistor in the pulmonary artery is measured. A temperature vs time thermal dilution curve is constructed. The area under the curve is computed by integration and this is inversely proportional to the cardiac output

Mixed venous oxygen saturation

- A fall in mixed venous oxygen saturation, in the absence of increased tissue oxygen consumption, is an indication of decreased cardiac output. Values greater than 60% generally imply satisfactory cardiac output while values below 40% suggest significant inadequacy of oxygen delivery

MISCELLANEOUS

ANAESTHESIA AT ALTITUDE

- Barometric pressure reduces with altitude; the percentage of oxygen remains constant (near 21%). The Po_2 therefore falls (see Table 1.4)

Table 1.4 Barometric pressure with altitude

Altitude	Barometric pressure (kPa)	Po_2 (kPa)
Sea level	101	21
5000 feet	83	17
10000 feet	69	14.5

The maximum P_AO_2 is limited by the presence of CO_2 and saturated water vapour.

$$P_AO_2 = (F_iO_2 \times \text{barometric pressure}) - \text{saturated vapour pressure of water* } - P_ACO_2)$$

- Reduction of P_aCO_2 by hyperventilation will increase the P_AO_2
- P_{N_2O} will also be reduced, limiting the efficacy of this agent at altitude (the need to give higher concentrations of O_2 will also limit the concentration of N_2O that can be administered)
- Minimum alveolar concentration (MAC) values of volatile agents are higher at altitude
- Vaporizers deliver a higher percentage of volatile agent (for a given setting) at altitude; however, this increase is in proportion to the reduction of pressure and the resulting partial pressure of volatile agent remains unchanged (saturated vapour pressure is essentially dependent only on temperature, not pressure)
- Flowmeters misread at altitude. In rotameters at low flow rates the gas remains laminar as it passes the bobbin, the pressure drop is thus predicted by Poiseuille's Law and viscosity is important. However, at higher flow rates turbulence ensues and density of the gas becomes important. Viscosity is temperature dependent while density is pressure (and thus altitude) dependent. Thus rotameters under-read at high flow rates at altitude
- Monitors of O_2 (paramagnetic, fuel cell, Clarke electrode), CO_2 (infrared absorption) read out as percentages although they measure partial pressure. Thus they read lower percentages at altitude although the concentration remains the same
- Temperature is generally lower at altitude (risk of hypothermia)

* Saturated vapour pressure of water at body temperature is approximately 6 kPa.

Altitude changes in the patient

- Hyperventilation
- Increased maximal breathing capacity (since air density lower)
- Acute pulmonary oedema of altitude or chronic pulmonary hypertension may occur
- Cerebral oedema or acid-base disturbance (acute)

Following adaptation
- Polycythaemia
- Increased red cell 2,3-DPG levels (shift to right of oxyhaemoglobin dissociation curve)

DAY SURGERY

Social factors

- Important to have nurse preassessment clinics to prepare patients and ensure their suitability, reduces cancellations and DNA rate
- Require responsible escort to and from hospital
- At home require:
  — Easy access to telephone (to facilitate contact should problems occur)
  — Easy access to toilet (particularly important following hernia and foot surgery)
  — Carer for first 24 h

Medical and surgical factors

- Duration of surgery now less important
- Patients with significant medical conditions should be excluded, including:
  — Uncontrolled hypertension
  — MI in past 6 months or severe uncontrolled angina
  — Muscle disease – myotonia dystrophica, other disease where normal activity is compromised
  — Severe respiratory condition such as uncontrolled asthma, severe COAD

Anaesthetic factors

- Requirement of rapid 'street fit' recovery
- No driving or alcohol consumption for 48 h
- Requirement for low incidence of nausea, motor block and postural effects limits techniques
- Procedures with delayed complications should be avoided (e.g. pneumothorax after supraclavicular approach to the brachial plexus)

- Patients must be clearly warned of potential complications and instructed as to who to contact in the event of complications occurring (a postoperative instruction card may be helpful)
- Postoperative pain should be minimized
- Multimodal approach to intraoperative and postoperative pain important:
  — Consider local anaesthesia, paracetamol, non-steroidal anti-inflammatory drugs (NSAIDs) and short-acting opioids
- Cases are short, therefore the number of cases tends to be large
- Recovery area with trained staff is essential

DENTAL ANAESTHESIA

General anaesthesia should be strictly limited to those patients and clinical situations in which local anaesthesia ± sedation is not an option.
Considerations as for day surgery, plus:

- Preassessment to be performed by referring dentist
- Clinical setting, must have:
  — Full monitoring
  — Resuscitation drugs
  — Spare apparatus (in the event of failure)
  — Dedicated anaesthetic assistant plus assistant for dentist
  — Appropriate recovery facilities, trained staff and monitoring
  — Protocols for dealing with patient collapse, resuscitation and transfer to hospital
- Competition for the airway between anaesthetist and surgeon (mouth not available for inhalation of anaesthetic agent – nose should be patent)
- Airway can become contaminated by blood; good packing essential
- Consider use of laryngeal mask and intubation where indicated
- Postural considerations:
  — Sitting with head slightly flexed – blood runs forwards out of pharynx but liability to postural hypotension
  — Supine – avoids postural hypotension but blood runs back into pharynx
  — Reclining with neck flexed to 90° – possible compromise
- Patients frequently exhibit severe anxiety prior to induction
- Dysrhythmias are common
- Frequently, numerous patients are treated at a single session
- Atmospheric pollution, particularly by N_2O, may be severe – consider total intravenous anaesthesia
- Beware of undiagnosed vasovagal collapse

Reference

Royal College of Anaesthetists 1999 Standards and guidelines for general anaesthesia for dentistry. Royal College of Anaesthetists, London

HYPERSENSITIVITY REACTIONS – ANAPHYLAXIS, ANAPHYLACTOID REACTION

Four classical types of immunological reaction

Type I   Anaphylactic (previous sensitization, immunoglobulin E (IgE) and mast-cell-mediated)
Type II   Cytotoxic (antibody-mediated)
Type III Immune complex
Type IV   Delayed hypersensitivity reaction

Anaphylactoid reaction

In addition 'anaphylactoid reaction' describes the clinical manifestation arising from non-anaphylactic histamine (and other vasoactive substances) release from basophils and mast cells.

Four types of reaction most frequently seen after IV drug administration

- Classical type I anaphylactic reaction (requires prior antigen exposure and specific IgE formation)
- Complement activation via the classical pathway (requires prior antigen exposure); C3 and C4 consumption seen, but generation of C3a results in levels < 30%
- Complement activation via the alternative pathway (C3 consumption with C3a production resulting in levels > 70% but C4 not significantly consumed)
- Chemical release of histamine and other vasoactive agents

Predisposition

- Increased incidence in females
- History of atopy
- No evidence of link to history of allergy and stress

Presentation

- Cardiovascular collapse – 90% of cases
- Bronchospasm – 50% of cases
- Generalized erythema or skin flushing

Management

Preoperative prevention in those at risk
- Anxiolytic premedication
- H_1- and H_2-receptor blockade

- Steroid
- Disodium cromoglicate

Management of reaction
- Follow normal A, B, C of resuscitation
- Remove any likely causal agent still being administered
- Oxygenate patient with 100% oxygen; intubate immediately if indicated (beware angio-oedema)
- Give adrenaline (epinephrine) IV (1 ml of 1 in 10 000 repeated every minute until satisfactory response)
- If no IV access give via ET tube (similar dose)
- Give fluids via IV line
- Consider use of steroids and antihistamines – beware: both can cause further vasodilation

Recommended anaesthetic agents (with a low incidence of association reactions)
- Etomidate
- Pancuronium
- Atracurium
- Fentanyl
- Volatile agents
- Regional techniques

Most common anaesthetic causal agents
- Suxamethonium
- Gelatins and dextrans
- Latex
- Althesin (now withdrawn)
- Tubocurare, alcuronium (now seldom used)

Reference

McKinnon R P, Wildsmith J A W 1995 Histaminoid reactions in anaesthesia. British Journal of Anaesthesia 74: 217–228

MONITORING OF NEUROMUSCULAR TRANSMISSION

Neuromuscular function can be assessed by

- Clinical observation (muscle tone, movement, respiratory movement, eye opening, tongue protrusion, head raising)
- Monitoring of the effect of nerve stimulation (visual, tactile, pressure transducer, EMG)

Reasons for monitoring

- There is marked individual variation in the degree of sensitivity to non-depolarizing neuromuscular blocking drugs

- Variation in the margin of sensitivity of the neuromuscular end plate (>75% of receptors require blockade before weakening occurs, 90% blockade is associated with total neuromuscular blockade; the dose-response is thus non-linear)
- The degree of reversal of neuromuscular block by anticholinergic drugs depends on the prior degree of block

Types of stimulus for neuromuscular monitoring

Single twitch
Supramaximal stimulus × 0.2 ms, no more frequent than every 6–10 s.

- Not reduced until 75% of receptors occupied
- Disappears when 90% of receptors occupied
- Twitch height < 5% of maximal will allow intubation and adequate abdominal relaxation for surgery
- Twitch height of 100% does not reliably indicate normal neuromuscular function

Tetany
50 Hz × 5 s, no more frequently than every 6–10 min.

- Painful: no fade indicates satisfactory recovery (equivalent to train-of-four (TOF) ratio of > 0.7)

Train-of-four (TOF)
Four supramaximal stimuli at 0.5 s intervals.

- Amplitude of fourth in relation to first gives the TOF ratio
- A ratio of > 0.7 indicates adequate clinical recovery
- Loss of fourth twitch – 75% of receptors occupied
- Loss of third twitch – 80% of receptors occupied
- Loss of second twitch – 90–95% of receptors occupied; this equates with adequate surgical relaxation

Post-tetanic count (PTC)
Tetanic stimulation (50 Hz for 5 s) followed by single twitch stimulation at 1 Hz.

- Allows assessment of profound blockade
- Relationship between number of single twitches present and speed of recovery to measureable TOF
- Speed of recovery related to specific relaxant

Uses of neuromuscular monitoring

- Facilitates titration of neuromuscular blocking drugs
- Avoids excess dose

- Avoids unexpected movement of patient or tightening (especially likely with shorter-acting agents)
- Permits use of muscle relaxants in sensitive patients (such as patients with myasthenia gravis)
- Monitors adequate reversal of neuromuscular blockade
- Helps determine cause of delayed recovery from anaesthesia or inadequate muscular power

Table 1.5 Features of depolarizing and non-depolarizing blocks

Depolarizing	Non-depolarizing
Reduction of twitch height	Reduction of twitch height
No fade of TOF* or tetany	Fade of TOF* and tetany
No post-tetanic facilitation	Post-tetanic facilitation

* Train-of-four.

References

Viby-Morgensen J 1982 Clinical assessment of neuromuscular transmission. British Journal of Anaesthesia 54: 209
Biebuyck J F 1992 Up and down regulation of skeletal muscle acetylcholine receptors. Anesthesiology 76: 822–843

TRANSURETHRAL PROSTATECTOMY

- Patients are frequently elderly, often with cardiac and respiratory disease
- Age and renal tract obstruction predispose to renal failure
- The lithotomy position limits diaphragmatic excursion with spontaneous respiration and increases intragastric pressure (especially in the obese)
- Water intoxication due to absorption if irrigation fluid from the prostatic bed (electrolyte disturbance, volume overload, haemolysis)
- Haemorrhage (may be difficult to evaluate with the large volume of irrigation fluid)
- Surgery can be prolonged
- Bacteraemia is common, especially where urine is infected preoperatively
- Hypothermia due to prolonged irrigation is possible unless fluid is warmed

Reference

Jensen V 1991 The TURP syndrome. Canadian Journal of Anaesthesia 1: 90–97

VOLATILE AGENTS

CHARACTERISTICS OF THE IDEAL VOLATILE AGENT

- Non-flammable; non-explosive
- Stable physical characteristics (no breakdown in light, not requiring thymol additive, non-reactive with soda lime, insoluble in rubber, non-reactive with metals)
- Appropriate volatility, giving low boiling point and high SVP
- Potent
- Safe (respiratory depression should precede cardiovascular collapse)
- Low blood gas solubility, giving rapid induction/recovery
- Analgesic
- Low incidence of nausea and vomiting
- Should not sensitize the myocardium to adrenaline (epinephrine)
- Non-irritant to the respiratory tract and pleasant-smelling
- Not metabolized
- Not hepatotoxic or nephrotoxic
- Non-teratogenic and not associated with abortion
- Without effect on the electroencephalogram (EEG)
- Without effect on CBF and intracranial pressure, or effect easily antagonized by hyperventilation
- Cheap

CURRENT AGENTS

DESFLURANE

Blood:gas	0.4
MAC	6
Boiling point	23°C
SVP	89 kPa

Advantages

- Stable (no reaction with light, metal, soda lime – for exception see below)
- Non-flammable
- Rapid recovery (low blood gas coefficient)
- Does not sensitize the myocardium to catecholamines as much as halothane
- Low metabolism (0.02%)
- Potentiation of muscle relaxants

- No increase in CBF and ICP if IPPV commenced at same time as its introduction

Disadvantages

- Pungent odour – unsuitable for gaseous induction
- Irritant to respiratory tract, particularly in concentrations > 6%
- Sympathomimetic effects – causes increased heart rate and blood pressure with rapid increases of inhaled concentration above 1 MAC
- Produces carbon monoxide when used with dry soda lime or Baralyme
- Low boiling point – requires special heated vaporizer
- Respiratory depressant

Reference

Eger E I 1995 Physicochemical properties and pharmacodynamics of desflurane. Anaesthesia 50 (suppl.): 3–8

ENFLURANE

Blood : gas	1.8
MAC	1.7
Boiling point	56°C
SVP	24

Advantages

- Non-flammable
- Non-irritant
- Does not sensitize the myocardium to catecholamines to the same extent as halothane
- Potentiates muscle relaxants

Disadvantages

- Pungent, not easily titrated for gaseous induction
- Associated with epileptiform spike and wave discharges on EEG monitoring (especially with high concentrations in association with hypocarbia)
- Occasional association with hepatitis
- Increases CBF and ICP
- Poor analgesic
- Potent respiratory depressant
- 2% metabolized (but free fluoride concentrations do not reach nephrotoxic levels)
- Produces carbon monoxide when used with dry soda lime or Baralyme

HALOTHANE

Blood:gas	2.3
MAC	0.75
Boiling point	50°C
SVP	33

Advantages

- Non-flammable
- Non-irritant, sweet odour (easy gaseous induction)
- Ease of titration during gas induction
- Bronchodilator
- Potentiates muscle relaxants

Disadvantages

- Sensitizes myocardium to adrenaline (epinephrine)
- Increases CBF and ICP
- Poor analgesic
- Potent myocardial depressant
- Requires thymol for stability (unstable in light)
- About 20% metabolized
- Relaxes uterine muscle (this can be an advantage on occasion)
- May cause idiosyncratic hepatitis, especially after repeated exposure over a short period

Reference

Ray D C, Drummond G B 1991 Halothane hepatitis. British Journal of Anaesthesia 67: 84–99

ISOFLURANE

Blood:gas	1.4
MAC	1.15
Boiling point	49°C
SVP	33

Advantages

- Stable (no reaction with light, metal, soda lime – for exception see below)
- Non-flammable
- Rapid induction and recovery (low blood gas coefficient)
- Does not sensitize the myocardium to catecholamines as much as halothane

- Low metabolism (0.2%)
- Potentiation of muscle relaxants
- No increase in CBF and ICP if IPPV commenced at same time as its introduction
- Hypotensive anaesthesia – dose-dependent reduction in systemic vascular resistance

Disadvantages

- Pungent odour, tricky when used for gaseous induction
- Respiratory depressant
- Produces carbon monoxide when used with dry soda lime or Baralyme

NITROUS OXIDE (N_2O)

Blood:gas	0.4
MAC	105
Boiling point	$-88°C$
Critical temperature	$36.5°C$

Advantages

- Non-explosive (but see below)
- Good analgesic
- Odourless
- Reduces the MAC of volatile agents by about 50% when 70% N_2O administered with O_2
- Low blood gas solubility so rapid induction and recovery
- No effect on smooth muscle
- Minimal effect on CBF

Disadvantages

- Weak (MAC = 105)
- Supports combustion better than O_2
- Diffuses more rapidly than N_2 (distends gas-filled cavities as it is 30 times more soluble than N_2)
- Diffusion hypoxia during recovery (Fink effect)
- Depresses marrow with prolonged exposure
- Pollution problem (more likely to be the cause of increased abortion risk than are volatile agents; not absorbed by charcoal)
- Difficulties of cylinder transport

SEVOFLURANE

Blood:gas	0.69

MAC	2.0
Boiling point	58.6°C
SVP	21.3

Advantages

- Non-flammable
- Rapid induction and recovery (low blood gas coefficient)
- Non-irritant, sweet odour (easy, titrateable gaseous induction)
- Does not sensitize the myocardium to catecholamines as much as halothane
- Potentiation of muscle relaxants
- Does not result in carbon monoxide production with dry soda lime

Disadvantages

- Relatively unstable, reacts with soda lime and Baralyme to produce 5 compounds (A–E)
- Reaction temperature dependant, worse with Baralyme
- Compound A (a vinyl ether) produced in clinical circumstances and is toxic to liver, renal and cerebral tissue in rats
- 5% metabolized in the liver, producing
  — Fluoride ions – currently does not appear to cause renal toxicity
  — Hexafluoroisopropanol – potential hepatotoxic, but cleared quickly and appears safe

Reference

Smith I, Nathanson M, White P F 1996 Sevoflurane – a long-awaited volatile anaesthetic. British Journal of Anaesthesia 76: 435–445

XENON

Only noble gas with anaesthetic properties at atmospheric pressure.

Blood : gas	0.14
MAC	71
Boiling point	−107.1°C
Critical temperature	16.6°C

Advantages

- Non-flammable, does not support combustion
- Lowest blood gas coefficient so rapid induction and recovery
- CVS stability (may reduce heart rate)
- Odourless and tasteless

- Chronic occupational exposure thought harmless
- Not environmentally damaging
- May be safe in MH

Disadvantages

- Diffuses freely through rubber
- Higher viscosity and density than N_2O may increase airway resistance
- Diffusion hypoxia during recovery (much less than N_2O)
- Increase CBF
- Infrared and ultraviolet absorption techniques cannot be used to measure concentration

HISTORICAL AGENTS

CHLOROFORM

Blood:gas	8.4
MAC	0.64
Boiling point	61°C
SVP	21

Advantages

- Non-flammable
- Potent
- Not irritant to the respiratory tract

Disadvantages

- Slow induction and recovery
- Sensitizes the myocardium to catecholamine (especially liable to provoke ventricular fibrillation during induction)
- Associated with hepatic toxicity (centrilobular hepatic necrosis)

CYCLOPROPANE

Blood:gas	0.46
MAC	9.2
Boiling point	−33°C
SVP	640

Advantages

- Rapid induction and recovery (low blood gas coefficient)

- Potent
- Not metabolized

Disadvantages

- Flammable and explosive
- Sensitizes the myocardium to catecholamine
- Marked respiratory depressant
- Nausea and vomiting

DIETHYL ETHER

Blood:gas	12
MAC	1.96
Boiling point	35°C
SVP	59

Advantages

- Does not sensitize the myocardium to catecholamines
- Cardiovascular stability during light anaesthesia

Disadvantages

- Inflammable
- Decomposed by light to acetaldehyde
- Pungent odour
- Slow induction and recovery
- Irritant to the respiratory tract
- High incidence of nausea and vomiting

METHOXYFLURANE

Blood:gas	12
MAC	0.16
Boiling point	105°C
SVP	3

Advantages

- Non-flammable at clinical concentrations
- Stable
- Potent
- Non-irritant; sweet fruity odour
- Good analgesic
- Does not sensitize myocardium to adrenaline (epinephrine)
- Little effect on smooth muscle

Disadvantages

- Extensive metabolism (> 30%) yields free fluoride ion which results in high output renal failure (2 MAC h is the suggested maximum continuous exposure)
- Very rubber-soluble
- Increases CBF and ICP
- Slow induction and recovery (high blood gas solubility)
- Low SVP so not normally possible to exceed an inspired concentration of 3–4%

TRICHLOROETHYLENE

Blood : gas	9
MAC	0.2
Boiling point	87°C
SVP	7.7

Advantages

- Non-flammable in clinical concentrations
- Non-irritant; pleasant odour
- Potent
- Analgesic

Disadvantages

- Sensitizes myocardium to adrenaline (epinephrine)
- Slow induction and recovery (high blood gas solubility)
- High incidence of nausea and vomiting on recovery
- Causes tachypnoea, but reduced alveolar ventilation results in hypercapnia
- Incompatible with soda lime; degeneration to dichloroacetylene (a cranial nerve poison) and phosgene in the presence of heat
- Smells similar to chloroform (waxoline blue dye added to trichloroethylene to differentiate it from chloroform)

ANATOMY

BONY ORBIT

Part of skull that contains the eye and its related structures, volume 30 ml. Walls can be thin and needle penetration is possible.
Irregular pyramidal shape (40–50 mm deep) with base forming the anterior opening.

Relations

- Superior:
  — Wall formed by orbital plate of frontal bone, lesser wing of sphenoid
  — Frontal air sinuses anteriorly, meninges and frontal lobe
- Inferior:
  — Wall formed by orbital plate of maxilla, zygomatic bone and palatine bone
  — Maxillary air sinus
- Lateral (45° to medial):
  — Wall formed by zygomatic bone, greater wing of sphenoid
  — Temporal fossa anteriorly, then middle cranial fossa, meninges and the temporal lobe
- Medial (parallel to the sagittal plane):
  — Wall formed by ethmoid, frontal bone, lacrimal and sphenoid bones
  — Nasal cavity anteriorly, ethmoid sinuses then sphenoid sinus posteriorly

Openings (Fig. 1.2)

- Optic canal – passage of optic nerve and ophthalmic artery from middle cranial fossa to orbit (see 3, Fig. 1.14)
- Superior orbital fissure – passage of lacrimal, frontal, trochlear, oculomotor, nasociliary and abducent nerves plus superior ophthalmic vein

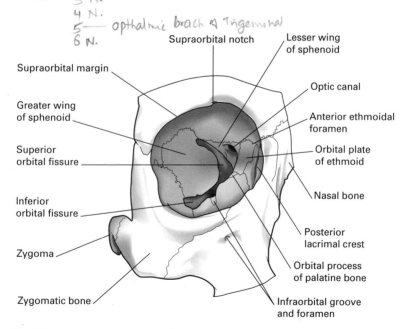

Fig. 1.2

- Annulus of Zinn divides the superior orbital fissure:
  — Trochlear, frontal and lacrimal nerves enter orbit outside the muscle cone
  — Area within the annulus is the oculomotor foramen
- Inferior orbital fissure – contains foramen rotundum allows passage of maxillary branch of trigeminal nerve (see p. 100)

EYE

Contained in the anterior part of the bony orbit, postioned nearer to the lateral and superior walls.

Axial length – distance from corneal surface to retina (> 26 mm denotes large eye).

Structure (Fig. 1.3)

- Anterior chamber   Area between the cornea and the lens, contains aqueous
- Choroid   Vascular layer between retina and sclera
- Conjunctiva   Clear membrane covering the sclera
- Sclera   Fibrous layer present around eye except in the cornea, 1 mm thick, thins to 0.6 mm at equator and 0.3 mm at insertions of rectus muscles

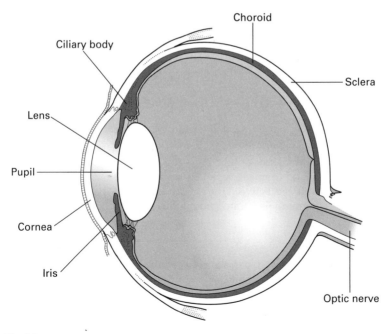

Fig. 1.3

- Cornea   Clear transparent outer coat of the eyeball
- Macula   Small area in the retina that provides most acute
                      vision
- Posterior chamber   Area behind iris but in front of lens
- Optic nerve   Enters through sclera posteriorly 1–2 mm medial to
                      and above posterior pole along with the central
                      retinal artery and vein
- Vitreous   Transparent, colourless gelatinous material that
                      fills eye behind the lens

Muscles

- Rectus muscles – superior, inferior, lateral and medial (these form the 'cone' within which lie the optic nerve, artery, vein and ciliary ganglion)
- Oblique muscles – superior and inferior

Innervation

Motor
- $LR_6(SO_4)_3$ – lateral rectus sixth cranial nerve, superior oblique by the fourth and the rest by the third

Sensory
- Trigeminal nerve (V) mainly ophthalmic branch, some maxillary

Blood supply
- Ophthalmic artery
    - — Main supply to eye and the orbital contents
    - — Branch of internal carotid
    - — Passes into orbit via optic canal inferolateral to optic nerve within meningeal sheath
    - — Pierces sheath to lie outside it when enters orbit
- Venous drainage
    - — Superior and inferior ophthalmic veins
- Important that no complete septal barriers have been demonstrated within the orbit and between the extraocular muscles – thus allowing local anaesthetics to penetrate through the cone

LARYNX

The part of the respiratory passage between the pharynx and the trachea.

The vocal folds form a sphincter protecting the inlet of the trachea and are important for phonation.

It is situated in the neck anterior to the laryngopharynx opposite C3–C6 in adults (see Fig. 1.4a).

(a)

C3—

Epiglottis
Hyoid bone
Thyrohyoid
membrane

C4—

Thyroid cartilage
Arytenoid
Cricothyroid
membrane

C6—

Cricoid cartilage

(b) Thyroid cartilage

Thyroid notch

Superior
cornu

Inferior
cornu

(c) Laryngoscopic view of larynx

Vallecula

Vocal fold
Pyriform fossa

Tubercle of epiglottis
Epiglottis
Aryepiglottic fold (false cord)
Cuneiform cartilage
Corniculate cartilage

(d) Cord movement

Arytenoids
pivot here

Posterior
cricoarytenoids

Lateral
cricoarytenoids

Interarytenoids

Thyroarytenoid

ABDUCT CORDS   ADDUCT CORDS   ADDUCT CORDS   RELAXES CORDS
(close rima glottidis)

(i) All innervated by recurrent laryngeal nerve.

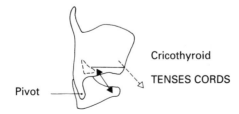

Cricothyroid

TENSES CORDS

Pivot

(ii) Innervated by external branch of superior laryngeal nerve.

Fig. 1.4

Structure

It is a fibrocartilaginous structure comprising six different cartilages:

- Epiglottis
- Thyroid
- Cricoid
- Arytenoid (× 2)
- Corniculate (× 2)
- Cuneiform (× 2)

Epiglottis
Likened to a leaf. Attached at its lower, tapering, end to the posterior surface of the anterior part of the thyroid cartilage.

Thyroid cartilage
Shield-like (see Fig. 1.4b).

Cricoid cartilage
Shaped like a signet ring (see Fig. 1.4a), articulates with the thyroid and arytenoid cartilage.

Arytenoids
Three-sided, pyramid-shaped, sit on and articulate with the cricoid. Adjust tension and position of the cords (see Fig. 1.4a).

Corniculate and cuneiform cartilages
Lie in the line of the aryepiglottic fold (false cord) adjacent to the arytenoid cartilage (see Fig. 1.4c).

Nerve supply

Supplied by two branches of the vagus:

- Superior laryngeal nerves
- Inferior laryngeal nerves (terminal branch of recurrent laryngeal nerve)

Superior laryngeal nerve
Arises from the vagus immediately below its inferior ganglion running obliquely downwards and forwards, crossing the greater cornu of the hyoid bone and thence along the outside of the thyrohyoid membrane. There it divides to an external branch (motor to the cricothyroid muscle and the inferior constrictor of the pharynx), and to the internal laryngeal nerve, which pierces the thyroid membrane to provide sensory innervation to the mucous membrane of the larynx above the vocal cords.

Inferior laryngeal nerve
Terminal branch of the recurrent laryngeal nerve. Supplies all the intrinsic laryngeal muscles (except cricothyroid) and sensation to the mucous membrane below the cords.

TRIGEMINAL NERVE

The trigeminal nerve originates on the ventrolateral aspect of the pons and passes forwards a short distance to synapse in the gasserian ganglion on the anterior aspect of the petrous temporal bone. From the ganglion originate the three divisions of the trigeminal nerve (ophthalmic, maxillary and mandibular) (see Fig. 1.8, below).

Ophthalmic branch

First division of the trigeminal nerve, entirely sensory. Runs forward from the gasserian ganglion (on the anterior surface of the petrous temporal bone) in the lateral wall of the cavernous sinus. Then enters the orbit through the superior orbital fissure and divides into three branches (lacrimal, frontal and nasociliary) (see Fig. 1.5).

Lacrimal
Sensory to lateral upper eyelid and conjunctiva. Also parasympathetic supply to lacrimal gland (parasympathetic fibres running via the sphenopalatine ganglion join from zygomatic branch of maxillary division of trigeminal).

Supra-orbital
Passes through supra-orbital notch. Sensory to upper eyelid, forehead and scalp (to vertex).

Supratrochlear
Sensory to medial upper eyelid, medial forehead and bridge of nose.

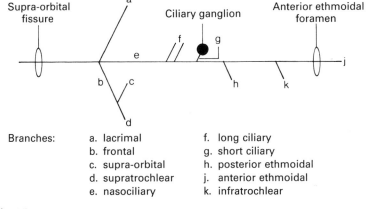

Fig. 1.5

Nasociliary
Runs on medial wall of the orbit to enter the anterior ethmoidal foramen (becoming the anterior ethmoidal nerve) to run on the cribriform plate through the anterior cranial fossa before running through the plate to enter the nasal cavity.

Long ciliary nerves (2)
Sensory to the eye. Also convey sympathetic fibres (from the carotid plexus) to the eye.

Short ciliary nerves
Run to the ciliary ganglion*. Sensory to the eye.

Posterior ethmoidal
Runs in the posterior ethmoidal foramen to reach the ethmoidal sinuses. Sensory to the mucosa of the posterior ethmoidal sinuses.

Anterior ethmoidal
Divides into septal and lateral branches. Sensory to anterior part of the nose and ala nasae.

Infratrochlear
Sensory to the skin of the side of the nose and the medial conjunctiva.

Maxillary branch

Second division of the trigeminal nerve (entirely sensory).

Runs forward from the gasserian ganglion in the lateral wall of the cavernous sinus and leaves the skull via the foramen rotundum to enter the pterygopalatine fossa.

The nerve continues in the infraorbital groove (as the infraorbital nerve) and then in the infraorbital canal, on the inferior aspect of the orbit and finally emerges from the infraorbital foramen (Fig. 1.6).

Meningeal branch
Sensory to the dura of the middle cranial fossa.

Zygomatic branch
Passes through the inferior orbital fissure to run along the lateral wall of the orbit. Divides into the zygomaticotemporal (sensory to temple) and zygomaticofacial branches (sensory to prominence of the cheek).†

* The ciliary ganglion also receives parasympathetic fibres from the oculomotor nerve and sympathetic fibres from the carotid plexus.
† Also transmit parasympathetic fibres from the sphenopalatine ganglion to the lacrimal branch of the ophthalmic division of the trigeminal nerve.

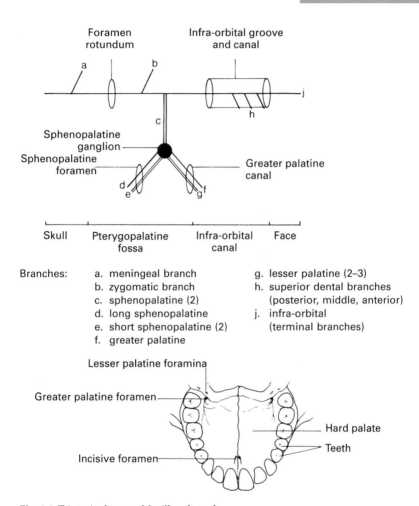

Fig. 1.6 Trigeminal nerve. Maxillary branch.

Sphenopalatine (2)
Sensory roots to the sphenopalatine ganglion (the sphenopalatine ganglion also receives parasympathetic innervation from the greater superficial petrosal nerve* and sympathetic innervation from the carotid plexus).

Long sphenopalatine
Runs through the sphenopalatine foramen to the roof of the nasal cavity then continues down the septum, finally passing through the incisive

* Originating from the facial (VII) nerve at the geniculate ganglion.

foramen. Sensory to anterior part of the nasal septum and anterior hard palate.

Short sphenopalatine (2)
Also pass through sphenopalatine foramen into the nose. Sensory to the superior and middle conchae and posterior septum.

Greater palatine
Runs though the greater palatine canal emerging at the posterior aspect of the hard palate from the greater palatine foramen. Sensory to the hard palate to the level of the canines and to the inferior concha of the nose.

Lesser palatine (2–3)
Also pass through greater palatine canal but emerge from the lesser palatine foramina. Sensory to soft palate and uvula. Small pharyngeal branches also originate from the sphenopalatine ganglion and transmit sensation from the nasopharyngeal mucosa.

Posterior superior dental nerve
Sensory to the upper molars and maxillary sinus.

Middle superior dental nerve
Sensory to upper premolars.

Anterior superior dental nerve
Sensory to upper canines and incisors.

Infraorbital nerve
Having emerged from the infraorbital foramen divides into multiple branches. Sensory to lower eyelid and conjunctiva, lower part of the side of the nose, upper lip and anterior part of the cheek.

Mandibular branch (Fig. 1.7)

Third and largest division of the trigeminal nerve, runs inferiorly from the gasserian ganglion. The only division with a motor component, supplying the muscles of mastication.

Nervus spinosus
Runs with middle meningeal artery. Sensory to the dura.

Nerve to medial pterygoid
Motor to medial pterygoid muscle.

Lingual nerve
Joins with the chorda tympani* and runs down beside the tongue around (below) Wharton's duct. Sensory to the anterior two-thirds of the tongue

---

* The chorda tympani conveys parasympathetic and taste fibres. It branches from the facial nerve.

Foramen
ovale

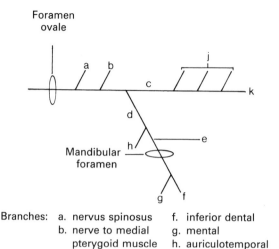

Branches:
a. nervus spinosus
b. nerve to medial pterygoid muscle
c. anterior trunk
d. posterior trunk
e. lingual
f. inferior dental
g. mental
h. auriculotemporal
j. nerves to masseter, temporalis and lateral pterygoid muscles
k. buccal

Fig. 1.7 Trigeminal nerve. Mandibular branch.

and floor of the mouth. Also conveys fibres from the chorda tympani to the salivary glands.

Inferior dental nerve
Enters the mandibular foramen to run in the mandibular canal. Sensory to lower teeth. Gives off the mental branch which emerges from the mental foramen and is sensory to the skin of the chin and mucous membrane of the lower lip.

Auriculotemporal nerve
Passes behind neck of the mandible to run with superficial temporal vessels. Sensory to ear and temporal region. Conveys autonomic and sensory fibres to the parotid gland.

Masseteric nerve
Motor to masseter muscle.

Deep temporal nerves (2–3)
Motor to temporal muscle.

Nerve to lateral pterygoid
Motor to lateral pterygoid muscle.

Buccal nerve
Sensory to skin and inner aspect (mucous membrane) of cheek.

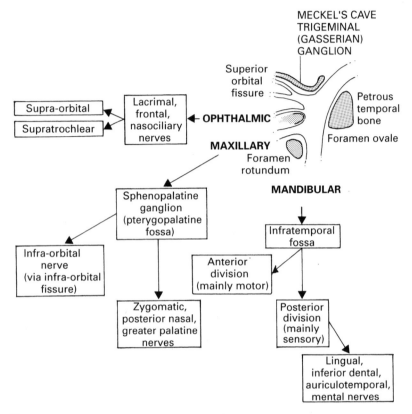

Fig. 1.8

DIAPHRAGM

Separates the thorax and abdomen. Peripheral muscle with central tendon which is continuous with fibrous pericardium above (Fig. 1.9).

Origins

• Crura (from vertebrae)
• Median arcuate ligament (joins the two crura)
• Medial arcuate ligament (over psoas muscle)
• Lateral arcuate ligament (over quadratus lumborum muscle to twelfth rib)

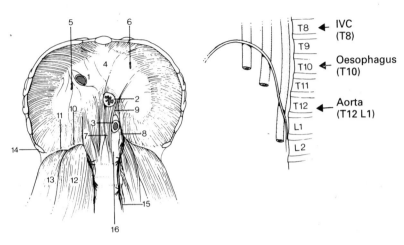

1. inferior vena cava (IVC)
2. oesophagus and vagi
3. aorta
4. central tendon
5. right phrenic nerve
6. left phrenic nerve
7. right crus
8. left crus

9. median arcuate ligament
10. medial arcuate ligament
11. lateral arcuate ligament
12. psoas muscle
13. quadratus lumborum muscle
14. twelfth rib
15. sympathetic chain
16. vertebral column (L2)

Fig. 1.9 Diaphragm viewed from below.

- Costal original (last six costal cartilages)
- Xiphisternum

Foramina

- Inferior vena cava (at T8 level in tendinous portion of diaphragm). Oesophagus and vagi (at T10 level in a sling of muscle mainly from right crus)
- Aorta, thoracic duct and azygous vein (at T12 level behind median arcuate ligament)

Nerves

Motor
- Phrenic nerves (C3, C4, C5)

Sensory
- Serous surfaces of central tendon innervated by phrenic (hence shoulder-referred pain from diaphragm)

- Peripheral (muscular) diaphragm sensation relayed via last six intercostal nerves

Excursion

- Diaphragmatic excursion 1.5 cm during quiet respiration, up to 10 cm with exertion

Embryology

The diaphragm is derived embryologically predominantly from three structures.

Septum transversum
Form central tendon; incomplete on each side leaving the pleural canals.

Pleuroperitoneal membranes
Close the pleural canals.

Muscular portions from thoracic myotomes to peripheral diaphragm

Congenital anomalies

- Most commonly failure of closure of the pleural canal (usually left) results in the continuity of the peritoneum and parietal pleura along the posterior body wall. Results in a congenital diaphragmatic hernia of Bochdalek
- Occasionally the muscular diaphragm may be defective (usually anteriorly). Results in a parasternal hernia of Morgagni

TRACHEA AND MAIN BRONCHI

- The trachea is 10 cm long in adults, extending from C6 level, and ends at the T4–T5 level at the carina where it divides into the two main bronchi
- The trachea is inclined backwards at 30° from the larynx to the carina
- The adult tracheal diameter is 1.5–2 cm and is flattened posteriorly
- Formed by fibrous tissue reinforced by 15–20 incomplete cartilaginous rings
- Lined by ciliated columnar epithelium and mucous glands
- Smooth muscle fibres are present posteriorly (both longitudinal and transverse)
- Right main bronchus is shorter (2.5 cm) than left, and leaves trachea at an angle of 25–30°
- Left main bronchus (5 cm) leaves trachea at angle of 45–50°
- Anterior relations of the trachea from above down include:
  — Skin and deep fascia

— Anterior jugular arch
— Overlapped by strap muscles
— Isthmus of the thyroid
— Pretracheal fascia
— Sternum and thymic remnant
— Brachiocephalic artery
— Left brachiocephalic vein
— Arch of the aorta
- Posterior relations include the oesophagus and recurrent laryngeal nerves
- Lateral relations include the carotid sheath and thyroid lobes in the neck
- In the chest on the right lie the pleura and lung with the superior vena cava
- On the left lies the lower part of the aortic arch

SEGMENTAL BRONCHI

The segmental bronchi are shown in Figure 1.10.

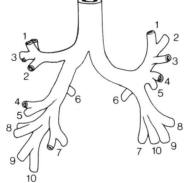

A Upper lobe
1. apical
2. anterior
3. posterior
B Middle lobe
4. medial
5. lateral
C Lower lobe
6. apical
7. medial basal
8. lateral basal
9. anterior basal
10. posterior basal

A Upper lobe
1. apical
2. posterior
3. anterior
B Lingula
4. superior
5. inferior
C Lower lobe
6. apical
7. medial basal
8. lateral basal
9. anterior basal
10. posterior basal

Note: Medial and lateral in right middle lobe and superior and inferior in the lingula on the left.

Fig. 1.10 Segmental bronchi.

Aspiration

- In the supine position tends to cause signs in the apical segments of the lower lobes
- In erect posture is most likely to enter right main bronchus
- In lateral position tends to enter upper lobe bronchus

Drainage

Drainage of the various lobes requires the positions listed in Table 1.6.

Table 1.6 Positions for drainage of lobes of bronchi

Upper lobe apical segment	Sitting upright
Upper lobe anterior segment	Supine
Upper lobe posterior segment	Lying half prone, half on side, affected side up
Middle lobe/lingula	Raise foot of bed 35°; supine, affected side slightly raised
Lower lobe	Raise foot of bed by 45°
Lower lobe apical segment	Prone
Lower lobe medial basal segment	Lying on side, affected side down
Lower lobe anterior basal segment	Supine
Lower lobe posterior basal segment	Prone
Lower lobe lateral basal segment	Lying on side, affected side up

FIRST RIB (Fig. 1.11)

- The shortest, flattest and most curvaceous of the ribs
- Runs forward at an angle of 60° to the spine and forms part of the boundary of the thoracic inlet (the first thoracic vertebra and the manubrium sternae form the remainder of the boundary)
- The tubercle articulates with the transverse process of T1
- The suprapleural membrane is a tough sheet of fibrous tissue which spreads over the cervical pleura and attaches to the transverse process of C7

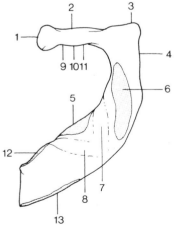

1. head
2. neck
3. tubercle
4. angle
5. scalene tubercle (area of attachment of scalenus anterior)
6. area of attachment of scalenus medius
7. groove for subclavian artery
8. groove for subclavian vein
9. site of sympathetic chain
10. superior intercostal vessels
11. branch of the anterior primary ramus of the first thoracic nerve running to the brachial plexus
12. area of attachment of suprapleural membrane (Sibson's fascia)
13. area of attachment of subclavius muscle

Fig. 1.11 First rib.

VERTEBRAE (Fig. 1.12)

- Each vertebra has an anterior cylindrical body and a posterior arch enclosing the vertebral foramen
- Contiguous vertebral foramina form the vertebral canal
- Each vertebral arch has a pair of pedicles and a pair of laminae and supports seven processes
  — One spinous process
  — Four articular processes
  — Two transverse processes
- The vertebrae are connected to each other by long ligaments (see below) and fibrocartilaginous discs between adjacent bodies

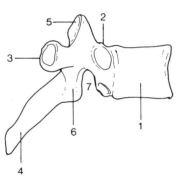
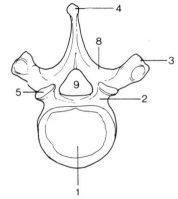

1. body
2. pedicle
3. transverse process
4. spinous process
5. superior articular process

6. inferior articular process
7. inferior vertebral notch
8. lamina
9. spinal foramen (forming the canal)

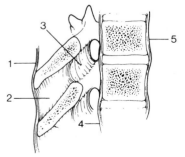
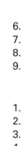

1. supraspinous ligament
2. interspinous ligament
3. ligamentum flavum
4. posterior intervertebral ligament
5. anterior intervertebral ligament

Fig. 1.12

- The intervertebral foramen is bounded by the inferior vertebral notch above, and the superior vertebral notch of the pedicle of the vertebra below forms the inferior boundary. Posteriorly is the capsule of the articular facet joint and anteriorly is the vertebra and disc
- The vertebral column has two primary curves (thoracic and pelvic) and two secondary or compensatory curves (cervical and lumbar)
- In the cervical vertebrae a foramen (foramen transversarium) is situated in the transverse process in which the vertebral artery runs
- The first cervical vertebra (atlas) has no body (but an anterior arch with which the odontoid peg articulates)
- The odontoid peg is situated on the second cervical vertebra (axis)
- The heads of ribs articulate with the bodies of thoracic vertebrae while the tubercles articulate with the transverse process

SACRUM (Fig. 1.13)

- Triangular-shaped bone, composed of the five fused sacral vertebrae

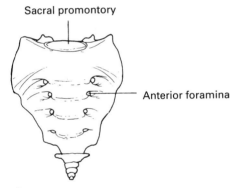

(a) Sacrum, anterior view

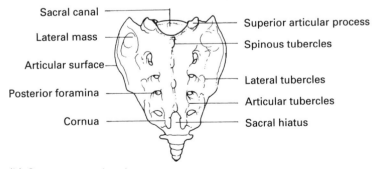

(b) Sacrum, posterior view

Fig. 1.13

- Articulates with the fifth lumbar vertebra at the base and with the ileum laterally
- The sacrum is curved with a concave pelvic surface
- The sacral canal runs dorsally, limited posteriorly by the fused sacral spinal processes
- The spinal processes of the fifth sacral vertebra remain unfused, leaving two sacral cornua with an arched opening (sacral hiatus) between. An elastic membrane covers the hiatus
- Pelvic sacral foramina open ventrally towards the ischiorectal fossa
- Dorsal sacral foramina open dorsally but are covered by multifidus and erector spinae muscles (which limits escape of injected local anaesthetic by this route)
- There is marked anatomical variation of the sacral canal which has important implications for caudal anaesthesia

Anatomical variations – implications for caudal anaesthesia

- The sacrospinal hiatus may be closed by bone, asymmetrical or widely open
- The distance from the sacral hiatus to the tip of the dura ranges from 1.5–7.5 cm. Indeed 2% of males and 0.3% of females have sacral spina bifida (i.e. the whole canal is open with no bony covering); in this situation high caudal injection is liable to result in dural puncture
- The volume of the canal varies from 12–65 ml (a fivefold difference)
- The size and patency of the foramina varies (of importance since injected anaesthetic solution, though blocked from flowing through the posterior foramina by the multifidus and sacrospinalis muscles, can be shown to escape from the anterior foramina)
- The lumbosacral angle varies from 7° up to 70° in patients with marked lordosis. Obstruction of cephalad flow of anaesthetic has been postulated in cases of acute angle
- The curvature varies greatly
- Such anatomical variation becomes more marked with age. Spread of caudally injected anaesthetic solution is predictable in children and clear anatomical features generally make injection easy. In adults spread is unpredictable

BASE OF SKULL (see Fig. 1.14)

1. The cribriform plate (through which pass the olfactory nerves)
2. The superior optic foramen (through which pass III, IV, VI and ophthalmic branch of V)
3. Optic foramen (through which pass the optic nerve and vessels)
4. Foramen rotundum (through which passes the maxillary branch of V)
5. Foramen ovale (through which passes the mandibular branch of V)
6. The foramen spinosum (through which passes the middle meningeal artery)

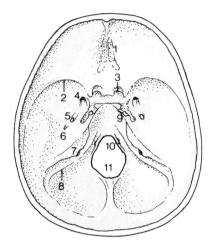

Fig. 1.14

7. Internal auditory meatus (through which passes the vestibular and auditory divisions of the VIII nerve and the VII nerve)
8. Jugular foramen (through which the jugular vein passes and which communicates with the sigmoid sinus superiorly)
9. Foramen lacerum (the internal carotid runs in the foramen lacerum but not through it)
10. The hypoglossal canal (through which runs the XII nerve)
11. The foramen magnum (through which passes the spinal cord)

SUBCLAVIAN VEIN (Fig. 1.15)

- Continuation of the axillary vein. Runs from the lateral border of the first rib, arches over the rib in the groove in front of the insertion of scalenus anterior to join the internal jugular behind the sternoclavicular joint
- The vein is most cephalad at the level of the midpoint of the clavicle
- Laterally it lies anteroinferior to the subclavian artery as it crosses the first rib. At the medial side of the first rib, scalenus anterior separates the vein from the artery
- Crosses in front of the phrenic nerve and costotransverse fascia (Sibson's) overlying pleura
- On the left side the thoracic duct passes behind the vein and enters at the junction of the subclavian and internal jugular veins
- The external jugular vein joins the subclavian vein after passing through the deep fascia above the clavicle

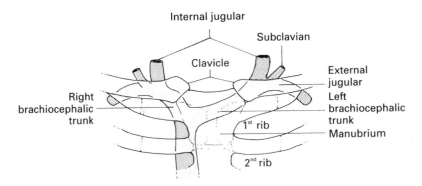

Fig. 1.15

INTERNAL JUGULAR VEIN (Fig. 1.15)

- Runs down the neck from its origin at the jugular foramen in the base of the skull (as a continuation of the sigmoid sinus) to terminate behind the sternoclavicular joint, where it joins the subclavian vein forming the brachiocephalic vein
- Lies lateral to the internal carotid artery in the upper neck and then the common carotid artery and lies in a common sheath with the vagus nerve between them. Deep cervical lymph nodes lie in close association to the internal jugular vein

Anterior relations (from above)

Lies quite superficially in the anterior triangle then deep to sternomastoid muscle, strap muscles of the neck and anterior jugular vein.

Posterior relations (from above down)

- The cervical sympathetic chain lies behind the vascular sheath
- Transverse process atlas
- Levator scapulae
- Scalenus medius (and nerve roots)
- Scalenus anterior (and phrenic nerve)
- First part of subclavian artery

BRACHIAL PLEXUS (Fig. 1.16)

- The brachial plexus is composed of the anterior primary rami of C5–T1
- Nerves emerge from the intervertebral foramina behind foramen transversarium (in which runs the vertebral artery) and between scalenus anterior and scalenus medius where the trunks are formed

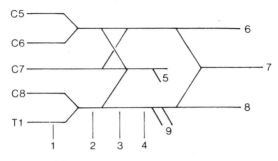

1. roots (5)
2. trunks (3) –
   upper, middle, lower
3. divisions (6)
4. cords (3) –
   lateral, medial, posterior

5. radial and circumflex nerves
6. musculocutaneous nerve
7. median nerve
8. ulnar nerve
9. medial cutaneous nerves
   (arm and forearm)

Fig. 1.16 Brachial plexus.

- Thence it passes across the base of the posterior triangle and over the first rib, at the lateral border of which each trunk forms an anterior and posterior division
- The divisions pass into the axilla in proximity to the axillary artery and form cords (lateral, medial and posterior according to their relationship to the artery)
- At the lateral border of pectoralis minor the lateral and medial cords give rise to the median nerve, while each also continues as the musculocutaneous and ulnar nerve respectively. The posterior cord continues to become the radial nerve
- Musculocutaneous and axillary nerves leave the sheath in the axilla before the lateral border of pectoralis minor

Nerves at the elbow

Ulnar
Runs on the posterior aspect of the medial humoral epicondyle.

Median
Runs medial to the brachial artery covered by the bicipital aponeurosis.

Radial and lateral cutaneous nerve of the forearm
Run together in the groove between biceps and brachioradialis (the lateral cutaneous nerve of the forearm is the sensory termination of the musculo-cutaneous nerve).

Nerves at the wrist

Ulnar
Divides to dorsal (sensory) and palmar (mixed) branches 5 cm proximal to wrist. The palmar branch runs medial to the ulnar artery and lateral to the tendon of flexor carpi ulnaris.

Median
Runs superficially in the midline of the wrist between the flexor tendons and the tendon of flexor carpi radialis, deep to palmaris longus (where this is present). Passes under the flexor retinaculum to enter the hand.

Radial
Passes deep to brachioradialis emerging (7 cm above the wrist) as several filaments that run superficially on the extensor surface of the lower arm.

Ulnar supplies

Motor
- Medial flexors of the wrist and fingers (flexor carpi ulnaris and medial part of flexor digitorum superficialis and flexor digitorum profundus)
- All intrinsic muscles of the hand save for the lateral two lumbricals and muscles of the thenar eminence

Sensory
- Little finger and medial aspect ring finger with medial aspect of the hand

Median supplies

Motor
- Lateral flexors of the wrist and hand (flexor carpi radialis, lateral part of flexor digitorum superficialis and flexor digitorum profundus)
- Pronator (pronator teres)
- Lateral two lumbricals and muscles of the thenar eminence

Sensory
- Lateral part of palm and thenar eminence
- Thumb, index and middle finger, with lateral half of ring finger

Radial supplies

Motor
- Extensors of the elbow, wrist and finger (triceps, extensor carpi radialis, extensor carpi ulnaris, extensor digitorum)
- Supinator

Sensory
- Radial aspect of the hand and lateral three and a half fingers (excluding tips)
- Posterolateral aspect of forearm and elbow

Musculocutaneous supplies

Motor
- Flexors of the elbow (biceps, brachialis)

Sensory
- Lateral aspect of the forearm (lateral cutaneous nerve of the forearm)

LUMBAR PLEXUS (Fig. 1.17)

- Anterior primary rami of L1–L4 combine to form the lumbar plexus
- It forms anterior to the transverse processes of the lumbar vertebrae with psoas major
- Nerves from the plexus are shown in Figure 1.17
- Nerves traverse the psoas muscle. The obturator emerges medially; the genitofemoral emerges on the anterior surface of the muscle; all the other nerves emerge laterally (to lie between psoas and iliac muscles)

Iliohypogastric

Pierces internal oblique muscle immediately above and medial to the anterior superior iliac spine to run deep to the external oblique muscle.

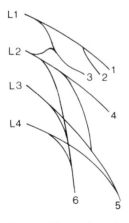

1. iliohypogastric L1
2. ilioinguinal L1
3. genitofemoral L1, 2
4. lateral cutaneous nerve of the thigh L2, 3, 4
5. femoral L2, 3, 4
6. obturator L2, 3, 4

Fig. 1.17 Nerves from the plexus include.

Ilioinguinal

Pierces the internal oblique muscle and traverses the inguinal canal in front of the spermatic cord.

Genitofemoral

Genital branch enters the spermatic cord at the internal ring and emerges from the external ring.
  Femoral branch passes under the inguinal ligament.

Femoral

Runs under the inguinal ligament in the femoral canal lateral to the artery and almost immediately breaks into numerous branches in the upper thigh.

Obturator

Passes round lateral wall of pelvis to run through superior part of the obturator foramen.

Lateral cutaneous nerve of the thigh

Passes below the lateral extremity of the inguinal ligament (1 cm medial to anterior superior iliac spine) and conveys sensation from the lateral thigh.

Iliohypogastric supplies

Sensory
• Suprapubic area and anterior part of side of buttock

Ilioinguinal supplies

Sensory
• Upper and medial thigh, ventral penis and upper scrotum (or mons pubis and upper labia)

Genitofemoral supplies

Motor
• Cremaster

Sensory
• Anterior scrotum and adjacent thigh (genital branch)
• Upper thigh below inguinal ligament (femoral branch)

Femoral supplies

Motor
- Anterior compartment thigh (quadratus femoris, sartorius)

Sensory
- Medial and anterior thigh
- Medial lower leg including malleolus (via saphenous nerve)

Obturator supplies

Motor
- Medial muscles of thigh (adductor magnus, adductor brevis, adductor longus, gracilis, pectineus)

Sensory
- Small area of medial aspect of knee

Lateral cutaneous nerve of the thigh supplies

Sensory
- Lateral thigh

SACRAL PLEXUS (Fig. 1.18)

Sciatic nerve

- Largest branch of sacral plexus, formed by anterior primary rami L4–S3 (anterior primary rami of sacral nerves emerge from anterior sacral foramina), which unite in front of piriformis
- Sciatic nerve leaves pelvis via greater sciatic notch running below piriformis and crosses the posterior aspect of the ischium on quadratus

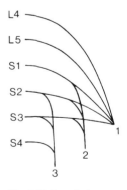

1. sciatic nerve (becoming tibial and common peroneal nerve)
2. posterior cutaneous nerve of the thigh
3. pudendal nerve

Fig. 1.18 Sacral plexus.

femoris (also obturator internus and gemelli) and adductor magnus. It
is covered by the gluteal muscles
• In the upper leg the sciatic nerve divides to form the tibial and
common peroneal nerves

Tibial nerve

• The larger division, runs medially to the posterior compartment of the
lower leg
• Gives a branch to the sural nerve and enters the foot behind the medial
malleolus, where it divides into medial and lateral plantar nerves

Common peroneal nerve

• Runs laterally and anteriorly curving round the lateral border of the
fibula. Gives a branch to the sural nerve and a lateral cutaneous branch
• Divides to form deep and superficial branches
• Deep branch enters the anterior compartment and terminates by
serving sensation of the first toe web
• Superficial branch remains in the lateral compartment and is sensory to
the dorsum of the foot (Fig. 1.19)

Posterior cutaneous nerve of the thigh

• Runs on the medial side of the sciatic nerve

Pudendal nerve

• Leaves pelvis via greater sciatic notch with sciatic nerve and behind the
sacrospinal ligament close to its attachment to the ischial spine
• Re-enters the pelvis and passes through the lateral ischiorectal space in
Alcock's canal (in obturator fascia)
• In the perineum divides into the inferior rectal nerve, perineal nerve
and dorsal nerve of the penis (clitoris)

Sciatic supplies

Motor
• Flexors of the knee (biceps femoris, semitendinosus,
semimembranosus) (shares supply to adductor magnus with obturator
nerve)

Tibial supplies

Motor
• Flexors of the ankle (gastrocnemius, soleus, popliteus)

Sensory
• Contribution to sural nerve

Common peroneal supplies

Motor
• Extensors of foot and toes (tibialis anterior, extensor hallucis longus, extensor digitorum longus) (Fig. 1.19)

Sensory
• Lateral lower leg
• Contribution to sural nerve

Pudendal supplies

Motor
• External anal sphincter (inferior rectal nerve)
• External urethral sphincter and anterior perineal muscles (perineal nerve)

Sensory
• Perianal, posterior scrotum (or labia) and dorsal aspect of penis (or clitoris)

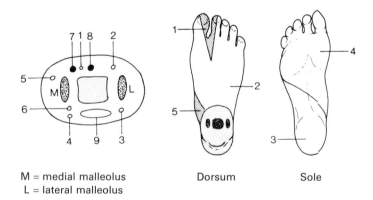

M = medial malleolus
L = lateral malleolus

Dorsum   Sole

1. deep peroneal nerve
2. superficial peroneal nerve
3. sural nerve
4. tibial nerve (becoming medial and lateral plantar nerves)
5. saphenous nerve
6. posterior tibial artery
7. tibialis anterior tendon
8. extensor hallucis longus tendon
9. Achilles tendon

Fig. 1.19 Nerves at the ankle and sensation in the foot.

Medial plantar supplies

- Similar distribution in the foot to median nerve in the hand

Lateral plantar supplies

- Similar distribution in the foot to ulnar nerve in the hand

INTERCOSTAL NERVES

- Each intercostal nerve is derived from anterior primary rami. Each runs segmentally under the respective rib
- The nerves emerge from the intervertebral foramina and pass through the paravertebral space (separated from the pleura only by the endothoracic fascia)
- The nerves reach the caudal margin of the rib at the angle and continue in the costal groove below the artery and between the internal and external intercostal muscles
- T1–T6 intercostal nerves are distributed exclusively to the thoracic wall, while those of T6–T12 continue down to innervate the abdominal wall (running between the internal oblique and transversus abdominis muscles)
- In the anterior axillary line a lateral cutaneous branch is given off and there is an anterior cutaneous branch near the sternum
- Each intercostal nerve serves sensation over a band-shaped area around the hemithorax (and abdomen in the case of the lower nerves)
- T4 (fourth intercostal nerve) innervates the area of the nipple, while T10 (the tenth intercostal nerve) innervates the umbilical area
- The intercostal nerves supply motor innervation to the intercostals, transversus thoracis and abdominal muscles

EPIDURAL SPACE

Boundaries

Above
Foramen magnum where the periosteal and spinal layers of dura fuse together.

Below
The sacrococcygeal membrane.

Anterior
The posterior longitudinal ligament covering the posterior aspect of the vertebral bodies and intervertebral discs.

Posterior
The anterior surface of the vertebral laminae and ligamentum flavum.

Laterally
The pedicles of the vertebrae and the intervertebral foramina.

Shape

Triangular in cross-section. The spinal cord and meninges lie within the space together with fat, the epidural venous plexus and lymphatics. The epidural space is widest in the midline posteriorly, in the lumbar region this averages 5 mm (however a midline septum and midline 'tenting' of the dura have been described in some patients).

Ligamentum flavum

Composed of elastic fibre disposed in a vertical direction. Thinnest in the cervical region and becoming thicker as it descends caudally.

SPINAL CORD (Fig. 1.20)

- 45 cm in length extending from medulla oblongata to its termination at the conus medullaris (at the L1/L2 level) from which the pia continues as the filum terminale
- Spinal dura terminates at the level of the body of S2
- 31 pairs of spinal nerves each with ventral and dorsal root
- Ventral and dorsal roots pass through the dura and epidural space independently and unite at the intervertebral foramina to form spinal nerve trunks
- Then divide into anterior and posterior primary rami
- Spinal cord terminates at the lower border of L3 in the newborn and at the lower border of L1 or upper border of L2 in the adult

Arterial supply

- Richest at cervical and lumbosacral enlargements
- Most tenuous in the mid thoracic region, i.e. it varies with the number of neuronal cells
- Major supply from the single anterior spinal artery – composite vessel made up of anastomosing segments of ascending and descending branches of the vertebral, intercostal and iliac arteries
- Contribution from the two posterior spinal arteries

Anterior spinal artery (Fig. 1.21)

Territory supplied by the anterior spinal artery is divided into three functionally distinct levels, each fed by one or more non-segmental nutrient arteries.

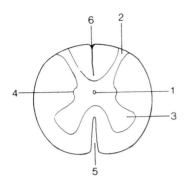

1. central canal
2. posterior horn
3. anterior horn
4. lateral horn
5. anterior median fissure
6. posterior median septum

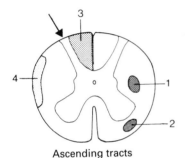

Ascending tracts

1. lateral spinothalamic tract
2. anterior spinothalamic tract
3. posterior columns (gracilis medially and cuneatus laterally–uncrossed)
4. spinocerebellar tract (uncrossed)

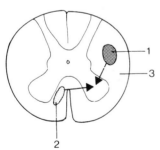

Descending tracts

1. pyramidal (corticospinal) tract (decussates in medulla)
2. anterior corticospinal tract (uncrossed, decussates at spinal level)
3. extrapyramidal tracts

Fig. 1.20 Spinal cord.

Cervicodorsal – supplies cord as far as T4
Small anastomotic arteries derived from the intracranial portions of the vertebral arteries descend in front of the cord to meet ascending branches from the subclavian artery.

Intermediate/midthoracic – supplies cord T4–T9
Small calibre of the midthoracic segments of the cord is matched by a meagre arterial supply usually arising from one of the intercostal arteries.

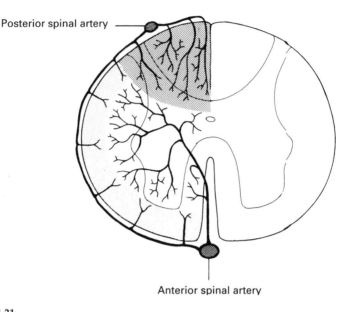

Fig. 1.21

Lumbosacral – below T9
Main supply comes from a single large vessel arising from one of the intercostal arteries (artery of Adamkiewicz – 'artery of the lumbosacral segment'). In 85% of cases this arises between T9 and L2. However, in the rest it has a high take off at T5 and is associated with an important contribution from the iliac arteries via the lateral sacral arteries.

Ischaemia

- End result depends on cause, duration and individual arterial anatomy
- In general most damage falls upon the territory of the anterior spinal artery
- Susceptibility increases caudally, is more marked in the anterior horns than the posterior and is more prominent deep within individual nuclei
- Effects of arterial hypotension can be exaggerated by coincidental rise in venous pressure

Epidural veins

- No valves
- Connect all segments of the body from pelvis to cranium by anastomotic linkages involving the caval and azygous systems

- Link to azygous vein via the intercostovertebral veins
- Lie mainly in the anterolateral part of epidural space
- Drain the cord and vertebral canal plus CSF from subarachnoid space
- Cranially communicate with the occipital, sigmoid and basilar brain sinuses
- Caudally communicate with inferior vena cava via anastomotic channels in sacral canal

Brown-Séquard syndrome

- Hemisection of the spinal cord results in the Brown-Séquard syndrome
- Muscular paralysis on the same side as the lesion and below it
- Vibration and position sense is lost on this same side also, while pain and temperature sensation is lost on the contralateral (unparalysed) side since the fibres decussate at the spinal level

PAIN PATHWAYS AND MODULATION (Fig. 1.22)

- Conveyed by small myelinated (A delta) and unmyelinated (C) fibres
- Synapse in dorsal horn of spinal cord (especially Rexed I, IV, V levels)
- Postsynaptic fibres pass anterior to the central canal to the contralateral ascending lateral spinothalamic tract
- Fibres in the lateral spinothalamic tract are laminated, with those from sacral levels running most laterally (fibres conveying tactile sensation run in the anterior spinothalamic tract)
- Fibres relay in the reticular system of the brain stem and run to the medial intralaminar and posterior nuclei of the thalamus and hence to the sensory cortex, limbus and hypothalamus
- Relay pain impulses in the posterior horn can be inhibited by mechanoreceptor stimulation (the 'gate theory'). In addition descending fibres can influence spinal pain transmission (e.g. the pathway from the periaqueductal grey matter via the dorsolateral funiculus). Both the periaqueductal grey matter and the dorsal horn of the spinal cord contain a high concentration of opioid receptors
- Evidence that above explanation is only part of the story, spinal cord is not 'hard-wired' in its functioning
- Pathways and connections are highly 'plastic' in their functioning so anatomical connections appear to be changeable

Conventional nociceptors

- High threshold nociceptive units found in skin, joints and viscera
- Polymodal activated by:
  — Moderately intense mechanical stimulation
  — Noxious heat and irritant chemicals
  — Joint receptors by movements outside normal range
  — Viscera receptors possibly to distension

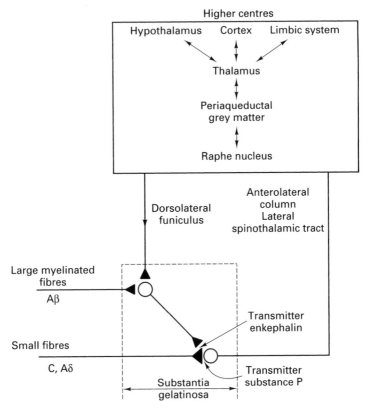

Fig. 1.22 Pain pathways and modulation.

Silent nociceptors

- Many C fibre afferents do not fire in response to any form of noxious stimulus
- In presence of inflammation they gradually become spontaneously active and mechanosensitive
- Inflamed area becomes tender and hurts on movement

Facilitation of passage of pain stimuli (spinal cord 'wind-up')

- Stimulus of C fibres at > 0.3 Hz leads to increasing length of discharge with each successive shock
- Excitatory amino acids such as glutamate are abundant in the spinal cord, released from both myelinated and unmyelinated fibres. Its effects are mediated by N-methyl-D-aspartate (NMDA) receptors and these have been shown to play an important role in persistent pain states. The NMDA receptor requires repeated and sustained stimulation by C

fibres for its activation. Once stimulated it leads to central hyperalgesia.
- Ketamine is a NMDA antagonist

Receptors

- Mu (μ), delta (δ) and kappa (κ) definite other subtypes controversial
- Opioid effects are mediated by several mechanisms but predominantly reduce neuronal firing. Presynaptic opioid receptors reduce the release of excitatory neurotransmitters involved in pain pathways. Postsynaptic receptors inhibit transmission by hyperpolarization
- Most spinal cord opioid receptors are located in the substantia gelatinosa. In the rat receptors predominate and 50% are presynaptic
- Cloning of receptors has brought new receptor that combines mu, delta and kappa structure. Known as the orphan opioid receptor (ORL). Opioid receptor ligands bind with very low affinity

Endogenous ligands

- These are the opioid peptides – three groups: enkephalins, endorphins and dynorphins
- In 1995 a heptadecapeptide was isolated and called orphanin FQ or nociceptin, closest relative is dynorphin. Superspinally it is hyperalgesic and spinally it is analgesic

AUTONOMIC NERVOUS SYSTEM

Sympathetic system (Fig. 1.23)

- Thoracolumbar outflow (T1–L3) from ventral roots of spinal cord
- Two-neurone system – ganglia present close to the spinal cord (sympathetic chain)
- Sympathetic chain extends from base of skull to the coccyx
- Preganglionic fibres short, myelinated – white rami communicantes
- Preganglionic transmitter is acetylcholine
- Ganglion mostly part of sympathetic chain exceptions:
  — Coeliac ganglion
  — Superior mesenteric ganglion
  — Inferior mesenteric ganglion
- Postganglionic fibres long, unmyelinated
- Transmitter noradrenaline (norepinephrine) exceptions include:
  — Sweat glands
  — Deep muscle vessels (both use acetylcholine)

Parasympathetic system

- Craniosacral outflow – cranial nerves 3, 7, 9, 10 plus S2, 3, 4
- Two-neurone system – ganglia mostly diffuse and near the organs they supply but four are well defined and associated with the cranial nerves:

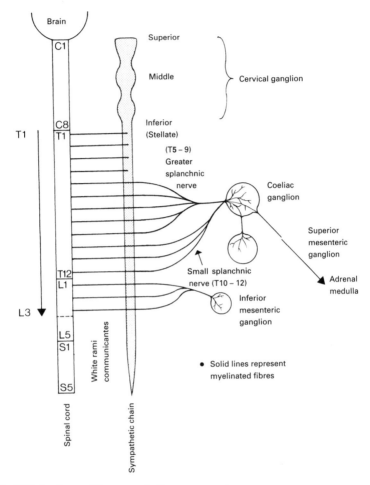

Fig. 1.23 Anatomy of the sympathetic nervous system.

— Ciliary ganglion
— Pterygopalatine ganglion
— Submandibular ganglion
— Otic ganglion
• Acetylcholine is transmitter at both preganglionic and postganglionic nerve endings but there are two different receptors:

Muscarinic
— Muscarine has little effect on autonomic ganglia but mimics acetylcholine at the nerve endings on smooth muscle and glands
— Blocked by atropine

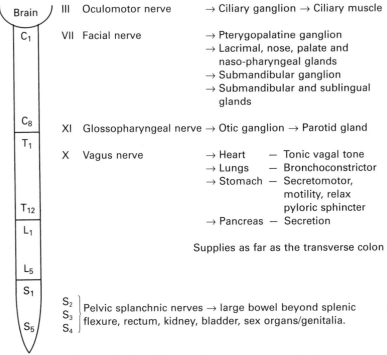

Brain	III	Oculomotor nerve	→ Ciliary ganglion → Ciliary muscle
C₁	VII	Facial nerve	→ Pterygopalatine ganglion → Lacrimal, nose, palate and naso-pharyngeal glands → Submandibular ganglion → Submandibular and sublingual glands

C_1

C_8 — XI Glossopharyngeal nerve → Otic ganglion → Parotid gland

T_1 — X Vagus nerve
→ Heart — Tonic vagal tone
→ Lungs — Bronchoconstrictor
→ Stomach — Secretomotor, motility, relax
T_{12} — pyloric sphincter
→ Pancreas — Secretion

L_1

Supplies as far as the transverse colon

L_5

S_1

S_5

$\left.\begin{array}{l} S_2 \\ S_3 \\ S_4 \end{array}\right\}$ Pelvic splanchnic nerves → large bowel beyond splenic flexure, rectum, kidney, bladder, sex organs/genitalia.

Pregangliomic fibres in both outflows end on short postganglionic neurones located on or near the visceral structures.

Fig. 1.24

Nicotinic
— Nicotine stimulates postganglionic fibres at the ganglia, like acetylcholine large amounts block transmission
— Actions unaffected by atropine
— These receptors found on motor end plate

REGIONAL ANAESTHESIA

GENERAL PRINCIPLES

- Local anaesthesia carries the risk of causing complications that may lead to loss of consciousness, the airway, convulsions or even cardiorespiratory arrest
- Same precautions as taken for general anaesthesia should be practised
- Patients should be visited preoperatively, be fasted and have their weight recorded

- History of problems with anaesthesia and local anaesthetics should be noted
- Procedure should be carefully explained
- Only perform where there are full facilities for resuscitation and trained assistance is available
- Equipment should include an oxygen supply, means of securing the airway and ventilating the patient plus suction equipment
- Drugs including thiopentone, suxamethonium, ephedrine and atropine should also be available
- Intravenous access should be established prior to performing a block and the same principles of monitoring applied as with general anaesthesia

Technique

- Skin should be carefully prepared for sterility after the landmarks for the block have been established
- When using alcohol-based solutions it is important to ensure the skin is dry before proceeding with the block; if using iodine-based solutions the operator should ensure that it is removed following insertion of block
- Decide on the volume and concentration of local agent to use and have it drawn up and ready
- Isolate local anaesthetic equipment and agents on a different surface to that used for other agents
- When paraesthesia has been elicited to determine the position of the regional block needle the operator should withdraw the needle 1–2 mm to avoid intraneural injection
- If the patient experiences severe pain during the injection it should be abandoned
- Aspiration prior to injection of the local agent is essential in an attempt to reduce the risk of intravascular injection.
- Use of the 'immobile needle' technique as described by Winnie (1969) is an advantage for many blocks
- Peripheral nerve blocks are slow in onset, particularly when using long-acting agents such as bupivacaine; therefore when using a regional technique as the sole anaesthetic the operator should allow considerable time (up to 45 min) for the block to become effective

Reference

Winnie A P 1969 An 'immobile' needle for nerve blocks. Anesthesiology 31: 577

NERVE STIMULATOR

Advantages

- Increased accuracy of placement of the regional block needle

- Unnecessary to elicit paraesthesia and so patient does not need to be awake
- If nerve stimulator provides an accurate indication of the stimulating current being used then optimal placement of the needle can be assured

Practical points

- Operator and assistant must be familiar with its operation
- Controls include a method for adjusting the stimulating current (ideally from below 0.5 mA to 10 mA); there may also be a means of adjusting the stimulus frequency
- Stimulus frequency should normally be set to 1 Hz
- The use of needles with an insulated shaft is preferred by many (this ensures the stimulating current is only emanating from the tip of the needle)
- When needle is some distance from the nerve a large stimulating current is used (in the range of 5–10 mA)
- As needle is advanced towards the nerve the appropriate muscle groups will be seen to contract rhythmically; these contractions increase in size as the needle is advanced closer to the nerve and the stimulating current should be reduced
- With the stimulating current set to 0.5 mA or less the needle should be finely adjusted to provide maximal movement
- Perform an aspiration test and then carefully inject the first 2 ml of the local anaesthetic agent. This serves two purposes:
  — It helps confirm the position of the needle as the muscle movement should stop as the nerve is pushed away from the needle tip by the local anaesthetic
  — If it is difficult to inject this suggests an intraneural injection and no further dose should be given until the needle is withdrawn slightly

INTRAVENOUS REGIONAL ANAESTHESIA – BIER'S BLOCK

Indications

- Most operations performed on the lower arm and hand; particularly useful for the reduction of forearm fractures
- May also be applied to the leg for foot surgery

Contraindications

- Sensitivity to local anaesthetic agents
- Requires the application of a tourniquet so should be avoided in patients who carry the sickle cell gene and those with severe Raynaud's disease

Drugs and dosage

- Preservative-free prilocaine agent of choice
- Low systemic toxicity and is available in 50 ml vials of 0.5% prilocaine
- Dose is about 40 ml for average adult (range of 20–50 ml ∝ weight of patient)
- Maximum dose permissible is 5 mg/kg

Equipment

- Suitable tourniquet:
  — Simple single cuff tourniquet with a pump and pressure gauge is recommended
  — If using double cuff systems or automatic systems utilizing air reservoirs the operator should ensure that he/she understands how the system works

Technique

- Follow general principles stated above
- Patient's blood pressure should be checked and noted
- Intravenous access should be established in the contralateral arm, then a 'butterfly' – type cannula should be placed on the dorsum of the arm to be anaesthetized
- Veins in the distal forearm can be used but the block tends to be more effective with more distal veins
- Upper arm should be covered with a layer of Velband and the tourniquet applied
- Prior to inflating the tourniquet the arm should be exsanguinated – if patient has a forearm fracture this is achieved by elevating the limb for 2 min while applying pressure to the brachial artery; otherwise the application of an Esmarch bandage ensures a more successful block
- Tourniquet is then inflated to 100 mmHg above the patients systolic blood pressure
- When satisfied that the tourniquet is satisfactorily in place then the appropriate dose of prilocaine is injected slowly over 2 min
- Block will usually be effective within 10–15 min and the tourniquet should not be released for at least 20 min after the injection
- The patient should then rest and be observed for at least 30 min

Examination points

- Technique brought into disrepute owing to several problems:
  — Use by staff untrained in resuscitation or with inadequate facilities
  — Use of inappropriate agents, e.g. strong solutions of bupivacaine
  — Tourniquet failures leading to toxicity

BRACHIAL PLEXUS BLOCK

Anatomy (see p. 109)

- Note that the musculocutaneous nerve leaves the plexus and enters coracobrachialis muscle high in the axilla
- Throughout its length the plexus lies within a tube of fibrous tissue which facilitates the proximal and distal spread of local anaesthetic injected at any level
- Sheath may have more than one compartment which may explain delayed or incomplete blocks seen with the various techniques of brachial plexus block

Indications

- Analgesia and anaesthesia over the arm; the choice of technique should be influenced by proposed surgery

Contraindications

- Allergy to local anaesthetic agents
- Infection over the site of injection
- Obesity and a short neck can make the interscalene approach difficult

Drugs and dosage

- Agent used will depend on the reason for its use
- If single anaesthetic and speed of onset is important then use lidocaine (lignocaine)
- If onset time is not important then consider prilocaine, lidocaine (lignocaine) or bupivacaine
- If postoperative analgesia is important then use bupivacaine
- Success of blocks is dependent upon the injection of a sufficient volume of local anaesthetic agent – at least 30–40 ml
- Use an appropriate concentration of the agent to stay within the maximum allowable dosage; in effect this means the use of 0.25% or 0.375% bupivacaine or 1% plain lidocaine (lignocaine) – 2% lidocaine (lignocaine) with adrenaline (epinephrine)

Equipment

- Short bevelled regional block needle, preferably 22 G – reduces the risk of damage to the plexus and allows the operator to develop a 'feel' for the characteristic click felt when passing through the sheath
- It is desirable to use the 'immobile needle' technique where a short extension set joins the needle to the syringe – provides stability once the needle has been inserted; an assistant should aspirate for blood and then inject the local anaesthetic
- IV access important

Approaches

- Interscalene and axillary approaches are dealt with here; others include:
  — Parascalene
  — Subclavian perivascular
  — Supraclavicular
  — Infraclavicular

Interscalene approach

- Effective for anaesthesia of the shoulder and lateral aspect of the forearm
- Ulnar aspect of the arm is less reliably blocked (in fact reliability of the block decreases as you pass up the ulnar aspect of the arm towards the axilla)
- Block is suitable for operations on the shoulder, lateral aspect of the arm, elbow and forearm

Axillary approach

- Effective for anaesthesia of the ulnar aspect of the forearm
- Lateral aspect and shoulder regions are less reliably blocked
- Block is suitable for forearm and hand surgery

Technique

Interscalene approach

Patient should be resting supine with the head tilted facing slightly away from the side to be blocked. The shoulder should also be gently depressed – it is important not to move the head or shoulder too far as this will make palpation of the landmarks difficult.

The cricoid cartilage should be palpated and a line drawn posteriorly from this some distance round the neck. The posterior border of the sternomastoid muscle should then be located at the level of this line (asking the patient to lift the head will help). Now ask the patient to relax; palpate at this point, move slowly laterally and a groove can be felt. The point where the line from the cricoid passes over this groove is the point of insertion of the needle.

With a finger placed in the groove just below this point the needle should be inserted at right angles to the skin in all planes. It should be slowly advanced in a slightly posterior direction until paraesthesiae are experienced by the patient. These should radiate down the lateral aspect of the arm: if paraesthesiae are felt in the shoulder then the needle should be repositioned. A 'click' may be felt as the needle passes through the facial sheath surrounding the plexus.

Following successful location of the needle and a negative aspiration test the neck should be gently compressed above the insertion point and the local agent injected slowly. The compression helps encourage the distal spread of the local anaesthetic.

Axillary approach

The patient should be positioned supine with a pillow positioned under the head so that the majority of its length is at the side the block is to be performed on. The patient's arm is then abducted to 90°, the elbow flexed and the shoulder rotated to allow the dorsum of the hand to rest on the pillow. Pain may limit this movement and, if it is difficult to feel the axillary artery, it may be necessary to lessen the degree of this extreme movement.

The axillary artery should be palpated and traced as high as possible in the axilla. The needle is inserted just superior to the artery and directed at an angle of 30° to the skin and kept parallel to the artery. The needle should be slowly advanced until the characteristic 'click' of passing through the sheath is felt.

Following a negative aspiration test the local agent is injected while pressure is maintained distal to the point of insertion. This helps ensure the required proximal spread to provide an effective block. A tourniquet applied to the upper arm prior to insertion of the needle is an easy way to provide the distal pressure, and has the advantage of reducing the amount of movement required of the operator once the needle is inserted into the sheath.

If the artery is punctured then this should be accepted as a useful landmark and the needle should be inserted through the artery so that it transfixes it. Then, after ensuring that the needle point has emerged from the posterior aspect of the artery (by performing an aspiration test), the local agent may be slowly injected. Following removal of the needle pressure should be maintained on the artery for at least 5 min.

EYE BLOCK

Eye blocks cannot be learned from textbooks, and the complications can be very serious for our patients. The candidate is urged to gain experience with a colleague who has extensive experience in this field and only use their technique. The following is only one of the many techniques in use.

Anatomy (see p. 89)

Globe and conjunctival block (block sensory components of trigeminal) is more easily achieved than akinesia (block of cranial nerves 3, 4 and 6).

Indications

- Anaesthesia for cataract and other eye surgery

Contraindications

- Allergy to local anaesthetic agents
- Infection over the site of injection
- Patient unable to lie still or cooperate during operation

- Open eye injury
- Axial length > 26 mm (relative contraindication)

Approaches

- Peribulbar
- Retrobulbar (Intracone) has a higher incidence of complications and will not be considered here

Drugs and dosage

- Various mixtures of local anaesthetics have been used including prilocaine, bupivacaine and lidocaine (lignocaine), though many now use 2% plain lidocaine (lignocaine) (± hyaluronidase)
- Peribulbar dose – 10 ml

Equipment

- 25 G 2.5 cm needle
- IV access important

Technique

- Conjunctiva should be anaesthetized with local anaesthetic drops (proxymetacaine then tetracaine (amethocaine) 1%). 10 ml syringe with lidocaine (lignocaine) 2% prepared. Patient lies supine and is asked to look directly ahead (providing something to look at on ceiling helps) so that eyes are in the neutral position. Two injections performed
- Inferolateral (aim to block ophthalmic branches – nasociliary, lacrimal, frontal, supraorbital and supratrochlear plus infraorbital from maxillary division)
- Palpate inferior orbital margin at its most lateral and inferior aspect, this is site for injection. It is useful to palpate and ballot the eye at this stage to gain an idea of its position. Insert needle either through conjunctiva or percutaneously with bevel facing towards the eye. Needle should be directed parallel to the orbital floor and lateral border of orbit. Contact with bony orbit may take place. When needle judged to have passed equator of the globe it is gently directed more medially (by 5–10°) towards the centre of the orbit. When hub of needle reached, aspirate and then inject 5 ml of the solution. Gently massage the eye for 5 min and assess block; if satisfactory proceed
- Nasal injection (aim to block medial parts of nasociliary, supraorbital and supratrochlear plus long ciliary and infratrochlear nerves)
- Ballot the nasal aspect of the eye. Insert needle (again with bevel facing towards globe) through the conjuctiva on the nasal side just medial to the caruncle. Direct the needle straight back parallel to the medial

orbital wall until hub is just protruding from conjuctiva. Aspirate and
then inject a further 5 ml of the solution. Again gently massage the eye
for 5–10 min and then assess block

Conclusion

Peribulbar blocks, though safer than the retrobulbar approach, nevertheless
have a significant risk of morbidity. It is possible to inject the local anaesthetic intravascularly or centrally. The globe may be perforated, and haemorrhage (retrobulbar and subconjuctival) may occur. Rarely the optic nerve
can also be damaged. More frequently though damage is caused to the
ocular muscles causing patients prolonged problems with double vision. In
view of this cataract surgery in particular is increasingly being performed
under topical anaesthesia

ULNAR NERVE BLOCK

Anatomy (see p. 110)

- The ulnar nerve arises from the medial cord of the brachial plexus at
  the lateral border of pectoralis minor
- At the elbow it crosses the medial head of triceps and lies in the ulnar
  nerve sulcus (in posterior aspect of the medial epicondyle)
- It then runs down the flexor compartment of the forearm and at a point
  5 cm proximal to the wrist it divides into dorsal (sensory) and palmar
  (mixed) branches
- The palmar branch lies medial to the ulnar artery and lateral to the
  tendon of flexor carpi ulnaris
- Supplies sensation to the little finger and medial aspect of the ring
  finger and hand

Indications

- Operations on the little finger or medial aspect of the hand
- In combination with median and radial nerve blocks for more extensive
  hand surgery

Contraindications

- Patients with ulnar nerve problems such as neuritis or symptoms of
  ulnar nerve entrapment
- Allergy to local anaesthetic agents
- Infection over the site of injection

Drugs and dosage

- Small volumes (5–10 ml) of local agent are required for this block

- Choose the agent and concentration according to the requirements for speed of onset and duration of action

Equipment

- 22 G regional block needle or standard 25 G needle

Technique

Two approaches, at the elbow and at the wrist.

Elbow approach
The arm should be flexed to 90° and held across the chest, then the nerve should be palpated 2–3 cm proximal to the medial epicondyle. The needle is inserted alongside the nerve and the agent injected. Injections to the nerve as it passes through the sulcus should be avoided as they have been reported to cause neuritis.

Wrist approach
The needle should be inserted at right-angles to the skin lateral to the tendon of flexor carpi ulnaris and medial to the ulnar artery. This should be performed at the level of the ulnar styloid process. 4 ml of local agent is injected if paraesthesiae are elicited, but injection of a larger volume (up to 10 ml) is usually successful in the absence of paraesthesiae. To block the dorsal branch it is necessary to infiltrate a ring of local agent (5 ml) around the medial aspect of the wrist.

Conclusion

Useful block to supplement inadequate brachial plexus anaesthesia or in combination with median and radial nerve blocks.

RADIAL NERVE BLOCK

Anatomy (see p. 110)

- Arises from the posterior cord of the brachial plexus
- Runs distally in the spiral groove around the posterolateral aspect of the humerus
- Continues anterior to the elbow joint with the lateral cutaneous nerve of the forearm to run in the groove between biceps and brachioradialis
- Passes deep to brachioradialis and emerges about 7 cm proximal to the wrist as several branches which run superficially on the extensor surface of the lower arm
- Supplies sensation to the radial aspect of the hand and lateral three and a half fingers (excluding tips) plus the posterolateral aspect of the forearm and elbow

Indications

• To supplement incomplete brachial plexus blocks

Contraindications

• Allergy to local anaesthetic agents
• Infection over the site of injection

Drugs and dosage

• 10 ml of the local agent of the operator's choice

Equipment

• 22 G regional block needle or standard 25 G needle

Technique

Two approaches, at the elbow and the wrist.

Elbow approach

The needle should be inserted medial to the brachioradialis muscle and lateral to the tendon of biceps. The needle will often be passed until it reaches the lateral epicondyle without eliciting paraesthesiae. The needle should be withdrawn 0.5 cm and 4 ml of local agent should then be injected, then a further 4 ml as the needle is withdrawn. This should be repeated with the needle tip directed more proximally. If paraesthesiae are elicited a single injection of 5 ml should suffice.

Wrist approach (simplest)

Inject a subcutaneous ring of local agent starting at the tendon of flexor carpi radialis, running around the radial aspect of the wrist at the level of the styloid process.

Conclusion

Useful to supplement incomplete brachial plexus blocks and when used with ulnar and median nerve blocks for hand surgery.

MEDIAN NERVE BLOCK

Anatomy (see p. 110)

• Median nerve arises from the lateral and medial cords of the brachial plexus at the lateral border of pectoralis minor

- Runs down the arm; at the elbow lies medial to the brachial artery and is covered by the bicipital aponeurosis
- Runs distally to lie in the midline of the wrist between the flexor tendons and the tendon of flexor carpi radialis, deep to palmaris longus (where this is present)
- Then passes under the flexor retinaculum to enter the hand
- Supplies the lateral part of the palm and thenar eminence, the thumb, index and middle finger plus the lateral half of the ring finger

Indications

- Used to supplement incomplete brachial plexus block or in combination with radial and ulnar nerve blocks for operations on the hand

Contraindications

- Allergy to local anaesthetic agents
- Infection over the site of injection
- Should not be used in cases of carpal tunnel syndrome or other forms of median nerve neuritis

Drugs and dosage

- Small volumes (5–6 ml) of local agent
- Operator should choose the agent and concentration according to the requirements for speed of onset and duration of action

Equipment

- 25 G needle, the standard disposable long-bevel needle being quite suitable

Technique

Two approaches, at the elbow and at the wrist.

Elbow approach
Palpate the brachial artery and insert the needle slowly just medial to it, adjust the position of the needle until paraesthesiae are elicited, then inject 5 ml of local agent.

Wrist approach
The needle should be inserted between the tendons of flexor palmaris longus and flexor carpi radialis muscles at the level of the proximal crease

on the wrist. The direction of the needle should be adjusted until paraesthesiae are elicited; then inject 5 ml of local agent.

Conclusion

Useful block to supplement inadequate brachial plexus anaesthesia or in combination with ulnar and radial nerve blocks for hand surgery.

ILIOHYPOGASTRIC, ILIOINGUINAL AND GENITOFEMORAL NERVE BLOCK

Anatomy (see p. 112)

- The iliohypogastric and ilioinguinal nerves are the first two branches of the lumbar plexus being formed from the anterior ramus of L1
- The genitofemoral nerve is formed from the rami of L1 and L2
- They form anterior to the transverse processes of the lumbar vertebrae within psoas major
- They traverse the psoas muscle and emerge laterally (iliohypogastric/ilioinguinal) or on its anterior surface (genitofemoral)
- The iliohypogastric nerve pierces the internal oblique muscle at a point about 1–2 fingerbreadths medial to the anterior superior iliac spine, then runs between internal and external oblique muscles running superior but parallel to the inguinal ligament, finally piercing the external oblique aponeurosis to supply the skin at the medial end of the inguinal ligament
- The ilioinguinal nerve pierces the internal oblique muscle a little lower and further medially and runs again parallel to the inguinal ligament before entering the inguinal canal to supply the scrotum/pubic area
- The genitofemoral nerve enters the inguinal canal and branches often supply the medial part of the groin

Indications

Blockade of these nerves can supply anaesthesia and postoperative analgesia for herniorrhaphy, orchidopexy and, when performed bilaterally, for Pfannenstiel incisions.

Contraindications

- Allergy to local anaesthetic agents
- Infection over the site of injection
- Presence of a pregnant uterus at or near term is a relative contraindication due to the risk of injecting local anaesthetic directly into the uterus
- Presence of an irreducible hernia may be a contraindication to the genitofemoral component of the block

Drugs and dosage

- Choice of agent used for this block will depend on the reason for its use
- If it is the sole anaesthesia for herniorrhaphy along with local infiltration then 0.5–1.0% prilocaine should be used, particularly in the poor-risk patient (volume up to 40 ml)
- If the block is being performed as part of a balanced anaesthetic then use bupivacaine 0.25–0.5% (20–30 ml is quite sufficient to provide perioperative and postoperative analgesia)

Equipment

- Short-bevelled regional block needle, preferably 22 G and at least 6 cm long. The use of this needle is important in this block as it allows the operator to develop a 'feel' for the characteristic click felt when passing through the aponeurosis of external oblique

Technique

Remember that the iliohypogastric and ilioinguinal nerves lie in close proximity between the internal and external oblique muscles.

The anterior superior iliac spine is the important landmark. The needle is inserted at the level of the spine and the width of one of the patient's fingers medial (the use of this size reminds the operator to reduce the distance in children). Once inserted perpendicularly through the skin the needle is advanced slowly until a click is felt as it passes through the aponeurosis of external oblique. It should then be pointed in a direction parallel to the inguinal ligament (towards the pubic tubercle) and the hub brought down to the level of the skin. The needle is then advanced just under the aponeurosis for a few centimetres. This ensures that the needle is advanced closer to where the ilioinguinal nerve pierces the internal oblique muscle.

10 ml of local anaesthetic is injected following a negative aspiration test. Following this the needle is withdrawn to the skin and a further 10 ml of local agent is injected superficially and through the aponeurosis in a fan shape. The genitofemoral block is achieved by inserting the needle one fingerbreadth above the pubic bone and injecting 10 ml of local in a fan shape into the superficial and deeper tissues.

Conclusion

Useful block that can be practised on anaesthetized patients and provides excellent analgesia following hernia surgery.

PENILE BLOCK

- Nerve supply of the penis comes from S2, 3, 4 via the terminal branch of the pudendal nerve, the dorsal nerve of the penis

- It passes along the inferior ramus of the pubis to run along the dorsum of the penis with the veins and arteries

Indications

- Operations such as circumcision or procedures on the glans

Contraindications

- Allergy to local anaesthetic agents
- Infection over the site of injection
- Adrenaline (epinephrine) should never be injected in the penis

Drugs and dosage

- Bupivacaine is the drug of choice for its duration of action
- Adrenaline-containing (epinephrine-containing) solutions should never be used
- Concentration and volume will depend on the age of the patient (in children the operator should calculate the maximum permissible dosage on the basis of 2 mg/kg and then choose the concentration depending on the volume needed)

Equipment

- 23 G or 25 G needle

Technique

Local agent should be injected to the skin on the dorsum of the penis at a point 2 cm from the base. The needle is then slowly advanced subcutaneously around both sides of the penis and further agent is injected ensuring that a complete ring of tissue around the shaft is infiltrated. It is useful to save 1–2 ml of the agent and inject this subcutaneously at the frenulum.

Conclusion

This is an easy and very effective block and avoids the side effects of caudal anaesthesia. It is, however, often easier for the surgeon to perform the block following the draping of the patient.

FEMORAL NERVE BLOCK

Anatomy (see p. 112)

- Largest branch of the lumbar plexus formed from the anterior primary rami of L2, 3, 4 within psoas major

- It emerges from the lateral aspect of psoas to lie between psoas and iliac muscles, then passes under the inguinal ligament lateral and posteriorly to the artery and almost immediately breaks into numerous branches in the upper thigh
- It is not present in the femoral sheath that surrounds the femoral vessels
- Therefore the sheath does not represent a useful landmark for femoral nerve blockade

Indications

- Provides analgesia over the anterior aspect of the thigh and the medial side of the calf down to the medial malleolus
- Provides analgesia for fractures of the upper femoral shaft
- It also provides branches to the knee joint; however, the sciatic nerve also provides innervation to the knee and femoral nerve block alone does not provide sufficient analgesia for knee surgery

Contraindications

- Allergy to local anaesthetic agents
- Infection over the site of injection

Drugs and dosage

- If speed of onset is important then use lidocaine (lignocaine) 1% with or without adrenaline (epinephrine)
- If onset time is not important then use bupivacaine 0.5%
- Volume required for this block is 10–20 ml depending on the accuracy of placement of the needle

Equipment

- Many texts only suggest the use of a short-bevelled regional block needle (preferably with an extension piece to allow the 'immobile needle' technique)
- However, the use of a nerve stimulator is to be recommended. Reasons for this are that the femoral nerve lies outside the femoral canal so this is an unreliable landmark; also the femoral nerve quickly forms anterior and posterior branches after passing under the inguinal ligament, making accurate placement of the local anaesthetic difficult. The accurate placement of the tip of the needle becomes more important for the three-in-one block (covered later)

Technique

Patient should be lying supine with the leg to be blocked slightly abducted. The initial landmarks are the anterior superior iliac spine and the pubic tubercle. These should be palpated and a line drawn between them: this marks the position of the inguinal ligament.

The femoral artery is then palpated and the needle is inserted 1 cm lateral to it and just below the line marking the ligament. The needle should be inclined so it is passing superiorly at an angle of 45° to the skin and directed towards the umbilicus. Often a click will be felt as the needle passes through fascia lata.

Once the patient feels paraesthesiae and following a negative aspiration test 10–15 ml of local anaesthetic should be injected. However, it can be difficult to locate the nerve and cause paraesthesiae; in this event 20 ml of local anaesthetic should be injected fanwise from the artery to a point 2–3 cm lateral to it.

When using a nerve stimulator the operator should look for contraction of the quadriceps causing movement of the patella. When this is elicited then 10–15 ml of the agent should be injected.

Conclusion

This block is probably much underutilized for pain relief following varicose vein surgery. However, it will affect the mobilization of the patient and, if the surgery is relatively minor (e.g. arthroscopy), then this should be borne in mind when considering this technique and the choice of drugs.

'THREE-IN-ONE' BLOCK

- The aim of this technique is to block the femoral, lateral cutaneous of thigh and obturator nerves
- These nerves arise from the anterior primary rami of L2, 3, 4, from within the substance of psoas muscle and then travel some distance in the same musculofascial plane

Indications

- Provides analgesia over the anterolateral aspect of the thigh, the medial aspect of the knee and the medial aspect of the calf down to the medial malleolus
- When used in combination with a sciatic nerve block it provides excellent analgesia for knee surgery
- Provides analgesia for femoral fractures

Contraindications

- Allergy to local anaesthetic agents
- Infection over the site of injection

Drugs and dosage

- Choice of drug and its concentration will be influenced by the volume necessary for success with this block as 30–40 ml of local agent are required
- Weaker solutions of bupivacaine (0.25–0.375%) may need to be used if this block is used in association with sciatic nerve blockade

Equipment and technique

Block should be performed as for a femoral nerve block. When the femoral nerve has been located and the needle is in optimal position the operator should occlude the area of the femoral canal distally using the thumb or fingers. The pressure should be maintained until after the injection has been completed. This pressure ensures that the local anaesthetic spreads proximally to the central musculo-fascial plane previously mentioned.

Conclusion

When assessing the success of this block the operator should test the lateral aspect of the thigh. If the lateral cutaneous nerve of the thigh has been successfully blocked then it can be assumed the obturator block has also been successful. This block can provide prolonged analgesia and affect mobilization following surgery. The femoral component in particular can last for longer than 24 h.

SCIATIC NERVE BLOCK

Anatomy (see p. 114)

- Largest branch of the sacral plexus being formed by the anterior rami of L4–S3 which unite in front of piriformis
- It leaves the pelvis via the greater sciatic notch running below piriformis and crosses the posterior aspect of the ischium on quadratus femoris and adductor magnus
- In the upper leg the sciatic nerve divides to form the tibial and common peroneal nerves

Indications

- Provision of analgesia of leg below knee except medial aspect to the medial malleolus
- Operations on the foot, particularly its medial aspect, e.g. Keller's osteotomy
- For knee surgery when used in conjunction with a three-in-one block

Contraindications

- Allergy to local anaesthetic agents
- Infection over the site of injection

Drugs and dosage

- 10–20 ml of local anaesthetic is required for this block
- Choice of drug will depend on the speed of onset and duration required

Equipment

- Short-bevelled regional block needle that is at least 10 cm long
- Use of the 'immobile needle' technique is preferable and so an extension piece should be utilized
- When using a nerve stimulator then a 22 G insulated regional block needle should be used

Approaches

- Can be approached by four well-described methods at the level of the hip joint
- Most consistently successful block is by the posterior approach

Posterior approach

This approach was popularized by Labat. The patient is positioned in the lateral position with the leg to be anaesthetized uppermost. The upper leg should be flexed to 90° at the hip and knee.

The position of the greater trochanter is established and marked by palpating the lateral aspect of the femur while holding the ankle and rotating the leg. The next landmark is the sacral hiatus. The final one is the posterior superior iliac spine. Two lines are then drawn from the greater trochanter, the first to the posterior superior iliac spine and the second to the sacral hiatus. From the midpoint of the first line a perpendicular is dropped and where this transects the second line is the point of insertion of the needle.

In the awake patient the skin should be cleansed and infiltrated with lidocaine (lignocaine). The regional block needle (e.g. a 9 cm 22 G spinal needle) is then inserted at right-angles to the skin and slowly advanced until paraesthesiae are elicited. To obtain the best success these should radiate down to the foot, then 10–20 ml of local anaesthetic is injected.

When using a nerve stimulator the anaesthetist should look for movement at the ankle (flexion and eversion). The volume of local agent required in this case can be 10–15 ml.

Conclusion

When assessing the success of this block the operator should test the medial aspect of the foot. This is a useful block for operations of the foot, particularly for painful bunion operations.

LATERAL CUTANEOUS NERVE OF THE THIGH BLOCK

- Arises from the anterior primary rami of L2, 3
- It travels downwards and forwards on the iliac muscle to pass under the inguinal ligament and into the thigh deep to the fascia lata
- At a point 10 cm distal to the superior iliac spine it pierces the fascia lata to supply the skin on the lateral aspect of the thigh

Indications

- Useful for anaesthetizing the donor area before skin grafting especially when used in combination with a femoral nerve block

Drugs and dosage

- 10 ml of the local anaesthetic
- Choice of drug will depend on the speed of onset and duration required

Contraindications

- Allergy to local anaesthetic agents
- Infection over the site of injection

Equipment

- Short-bevelled regional block needle

Technique

The important landmark is the anterior superior iliac spine. This is palpated and marked on the supine patient. The needle should be inserted perpendicularly at a point 1 cm medial and 2 cm inferior to the spine. The needle should be slowly advanced until a click is felt as it passes through fascia lata. Following a negative aspiration test 2–4 ml of the local agent is injected. The needle is then withdrawn to just below the skin and the process repeated in a fanwise fashion until a total of 10 ml has been injected below the fascia.

Conclusion

This is an easy block to perform and become proficient at, and it has the advantage of familiarizing the operator with the characteristic feel of passing the needle through a ligamentous tissue plane. This feel is important for success in both iliohypogastric and axillary plexus blocks.

CAUDAL ANAESTHESIA

- Injection of local anaesthetic agent via the sacral hiatus into the sacral canal is termed a 'caudal' in regional anaesthesia
- One of the first reported approaches to the epidural space and, if its limitations are understood, can still be useful in modern anaesthetic practice

Anatomy

See page 106.

Indications

- *Paediatrics*: this block is useful for analgesia following orchidopexy, herniorrhaphy, penile and foot surgery
- *Adults*: useful for operations on the genitalia, the perineum, the prostate, haemorrhoids and operations on the feet such as Keller's osteotomy

Contraindications

- Bleeding diathesis
- Allergy to local anaesthetic agents
- Infection over the site of injection
- Has been used successfully in obstetrics to provide analgesia for forceps deliveries but this should only be undertaken by those experienced with the technique because of the risk of injecting the local agent into the head of the fetus

Drugs and dosage

- Bupivacaine is the drug of choice to provide maximal duration of analgesia
- Using sufficient volume is the secret of success, and in paediatric practice the volume required will depend on the height of block desired
- For orchidopexy and hernia surgery a large volume of agent is necessary. In this situation it is safest to calculate the maximum dosage for the patient and then calculate the volume required based on the formula of 0.1 ml of bupivacaine per segment to be blocked per year of age of the child (therefore necessary to use the 0.25% solution in younger age groups)
- In adults the dose is 15–20 ml of 0.25–0.5% bupivacaine

Equipment

- Operator should prepare for this block as for a single-shot epidural
- Use of a regional block tray, skin preparation solution and a filter needle to draw up the solution are recommended
- Standard 21 G disposable hypodermic needle is satisfactory for adults but a 22 G regional block needle will provide more feel and this should be used in children

Technique

Classically the patient should be placed in the prone position with a pillow under the symphysis pubis. However, if using this block in association with a general anaesthetic it is easier to perform with the patient in the left lateral position. The knees are flexed and the legs brought up to lie at right-angles to the spine.

The operator should then palpate for the sacral hiatus using the sacral cornua as a landmark. If the hiatus is not obvious then the operator can palpate and mark the posterior superior iliac spines and then join these with a line. This forms the base of an equilateral triangle (pointing caudally) with its apex at the sacral hiatus.

Having established the position of the sacral hiatus the operator should prepare the skin and proceed. The needle should be inserted just caudally to the sacral cornua at an angle of 45°. A click should be felt as it passes through the membrane covering the hiatus.

The operator should then aspirate on the syringe, then slowly inject the local agent. Because of the variable distance between the sacral hiatus and the dura the practice of advancing the needle up the sacral canal prior to injecting the local agent cannot be recommended.

Conclusion

This block is ideal for transurethral prostatectomies as it provides good per- and postoperative analgesia. It should also be considered in orthopaedics when the surgeon is performing bilateral foot surgery.

INTERCOSTAL BLOCK

Anatomy

See page 117.

Indications

- Provision of analgesia for fractured ribs
- Operations involving unilateral abdominal incisions – cholecystectomy, splenectomy
- Bilateral blocks can provide analgesia for midline incisions

Contraindications

- Allergy to local anaesthetic agents
- Infection over the site of injection

Drugs and dosage

- Bupivacaine is the drug of choice to provide maximal duration of analgesia
- Volume and concentration are dependent on number of ribs to be blocked (normal dose 5 ml of 0.5% per rib)

Equipment

- 22 G regional block needle is preferred but standard 21 G disposable hypodermic needle is satisfactory

Technique

The patient should be sitting up or be in the lateral position (side to be blocked uppermost). The arms should be held forward and the shoulders abducted to move the scapulae laterally allowing access to the posterior aspect of the ribs. The ribs should be palpated as posteriorly as possible (between the posterior rib angles and the posterior axillary line) and those to be blocked marked.

The needle is inserted perpendicular to the skin and passed on to the rib, then the needle is gradually moved down the rib until it can pass just inferior to it. The needle should be inserted for 2–3 mm and the syringe should be aspirated before injection of the local agent.

Conclusion

Useful block for postoperative analgesia following cholecystectomy. Risk of causing pneumothorax, so bilateral blocks should only be performed by the very experienced operator.

Table 1.7 suggests volumes and concentrations of drug to use for various blocks (based on the average adult). Examples of operations the block may be suitable for are included.

Table 1.7 Drug volumes and concentrations for regional anaesthesia

Block	Drug/dosage	Operation
Bier's	Prilocaine 0.5% 40 ml	Colles fracture Carpal tunnel

Interscalene	Prilocaine 1% 30–40 ml
	Lidocaine (lignocaine) 1%
	    30–40 ml with adrenaline
	    (epinephrine)
	Bupivacaine 0.25% 40 ml
	Bupivacaine 0.5% 30 ml
		Shoulder, upper arm, elbow,
		    forearm or hand. Beware
		    deficient analgesia on ulnar
		    aspect

Axillary	As above	Forearm and hand surgery,
		    insertion of vascular shunts.
		    Beware deficient analgesia on
		    lateral aspect of arm

Median	Lidocaine (lignocaine) 1%
	    6 ml
	Bupivacaine 0.5% 6 ml
		Usually only used with radial
		    and ulnar blocks for hand
		    surgery. Useful to supplement
		    incomplete brachial block

Radial	Lidocaine (lignocaine) 1% 10 ml Bupivacaine 0.5% 10 ml	See above

Ulnar	Lidocaine (lignocaine) 1%
	    6 ml
	Bupivacaine 0.5% 6 ml
		Operations on little finger,
		    fifth metacarpal

Intercostal	Bupivacaine 0.5% 5 ml	Following unilateral
		    abdominal incisions –
		    cholecystectomy, splenectomy

Ilioinguinal
Ioliohypogastric
Genitofemoral
	Lidocaine (lignocaine) 1%
	    30 ml with adrenaline
	    (epinephrine)
	Prilocaine 0.5% 30 ml
	Bupivacaine 0.5% 20 ml
		Inguinal herniorrhaphy, can
		    use bilaterally for analgesia
		    following Pfannenstiel
		    incision

Caudal	Bupivacaine 0.5% 20 ml	Haemorrhoids and other anal
		    surgery, TURP, penile and
		    perineal surgery

Penile	Bupivacaine 0.5% 10–15 ml	Circumcision

Femoral	Bupivacaine 0.5% 10 ml
	Lidocaine (lignocaine) 1%
	    10 ml with adrenaline
	    (epinephrine)
		Femoral shaft fractures

Three-in-one	Bupivacaine 0.25% 30 ml
	Lidocaine (lignocaine) 1%
	    30 ml with adrenaline
	    (epinephrine)
		Femoral shaft fractures, skin
		    grafting from thigh, knee
		    surgery

Sciatic	Bupivacaine 0.5% 15 ml	In conjunction with three-in-
		    one block for knee
		    replacement, foot surgery

Practical clinical section

Electrocardiograms (ECGs) chest X-rays, pulmonary function tests and blood gas interpretation are fundamental to normal anaesthetic clinical practice and consequently feature significantly in examinations. Candidates should demonstrate a thorough knowledge and understanding of these fields.

The following sections are intended for use primarily as synopses. Candidates are strongly recommended to consult more comprehensive specific texts. Specialists in each field (physicians, cardiologists, radiologists, etc.) are available in every hospital and wherever possible candidates should turn to them for supplementary teaching.

ECG

INTERPRETATION OF THE ELECTROCARDIOGRAM (ECG)

Electrocardiograms (ECGs) are frequently encountered in clinical anaesthetic exams and competent interpretation is expected. ECGs are performed every day in patients before surgery and failure of a candidate to report potentially dangerous features correctly suggests that the candidate is unsafe and he/she is likely to be failed. The ECG should be approached in a systematic way, even when obvious abnormalities are instantly apparent; there are often multiple abnormalities on a single ECG (especially in exams). The candidate should develop a system for ECG interpretation and practise using this on the ward when confronted by ECGs; in this way the system should become second nature.

A suggested system for basic ECG interpretation

1. *Check the name and age of the patient*
   Where is this stated?

2. *Check the gain*
   10 mm/mV is normal and a 1 mV standard should be included.
   Particularly check that no leads (especially lateral chest leads) are
   recorded at half voltage.

3. *Check the recording rate*
   Normal rate is 25 mm/s; 50 mm/s can also be employed.

4. *Determine whether the patient is in sinus rhythm*
   If not, is the rhythm regular or irregular?

5. *Determine the heart rate*
   Each small square is 0.04 s and each large square 0.2 s at normal rate
   (25 mm/s).
   Rapid approximation of the rate can be made by counting the number
   of large squares between adjacent R waves:
   Rate = 300/number of large squares.

6. *Evaluate the P waves*
   a. The P wave should be less than three small squares in width and
      2.5 mm in height in lead II.
   b. The P wave in lead V1 should be predominantly positive.

7. *Check the P-R interval*
   The P-R interval (measured from the start of the P wave to the start of
   the QRS complex) should be shorter than 0.2 (five small squares)
   and longer than 0.12 s (three small squares).

8. *Check the QRS complexes*
   a. *Measure the QRS duration:* should not exceed 0.10 s (two small
      squares)
   b. *Look for abnormal Q waves:* any Q wave should not equal or exceed
      0.04 s duration and should be less than one-quarter of the ensuing
      T wave in depth – except in leads III and AVR, which look into the
      heart cavity (also AVL when the frontal plane axis is more positive
      than +60%), and where such Q waves can occur without being
      abnormal
   c. *Check smooth R wave progression in chest leads:* there should be a
      smooth increase in the R wave height across the chest leads
      (Fig. 2.1a), although smooth diminution of the R wave in V5 and
      V6 is permissible (Fig. 2.1b). At least one R wave in the chest leads
      should exceed 8 mm in height
   d. *Check R and S wave dimensions:*
      — in the chest leads the tallest R wave should not exceed 30 mm;
        in the chest leads the deepest S wave should not exceed 30 mm;
        the sum of the tallest R and deepest S wave in the chest leads
        should not exceed 40 mm
      — the ventricular activation time (start of QRS to maximum R
        wave) should not exceed 0.04 s
      — in the limb leads the R wave in AVL should be less than 15 mm
        and that in AVF less than 20 mm

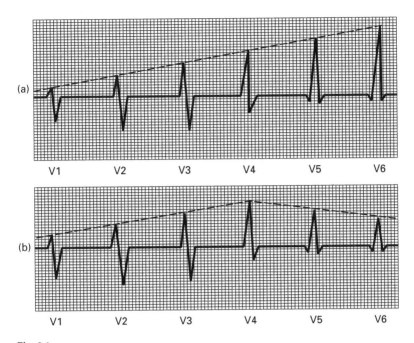

Fig. 2.1

e. *Calculate the mean frontal plane axis:* the mean frontal plane axis should be between −30° and +90°; the frontal axis is calculated with regard to the relative positions from which the limb leads look at the heart. A diagrammatic representation of these positions is shown in Figure 2.2a. The most isoelectric lead should be identified; that is the lead where the R and S waves are of equal magnitude and R − S = O (so lead I is isoelectric in Fig. 2.2b). The axis will be at right angles to this lead so in this example will be either at +90° (towards AVF) or at −90° (between AVL and AVR). It can be readily appreciated that AVF is more positive while AVL and AVR are predominantly negative; the axis is therefore about +90° (Fig. 2.2b). Finally the two leads each side of the most positive lead should be examined (II and III in Fig. 2.2c). If one is more positive than the other, then the axis will be slightly towards this (in the example II is more positive than III so the axis is a little less than +90°, i.e. it is normal).

9. *Look at the S-T segments:* the S-T segments should not deviate from the isoelectric line (baseline) by more than 1 mm (either above or below). Rapid tachycardia may make assessment of the S-T segments very difficult.

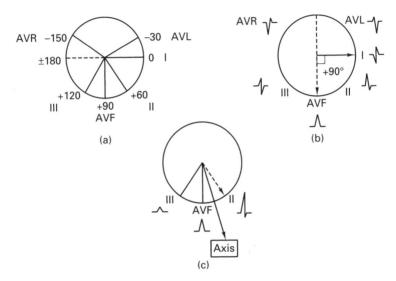

Fig. 2.2

10. *Look at the T waves:*
    a. The T wave in V3–V6 should be upright. The T wave in V1 and V2 should be upright if this was the case in previous records
    b. In the limb leads the T wave axis should be within 45° of the QRS axis

SUMMARY OF SYSTEMATIC ECG INTERPRETATION

1. Name, age
2. Gain (voltage)
3. Recording rate
4. Rhythm
5. Rate
6. P waves
7. P-R interval
8. QRS complexes:
   a. QRS duration
   b. abnormal Q waves
   c. smooth R wave progression in chest leads
   d. R and S wave dimensions
   e. mean frontal plane axis
9. S-T segment
10. T waves

SPECIFIC CRITERIA FOR ECG DIAGNOSIS

Left atrial enlargement

- P wave duration of > 0.12 s
- Bifid P wave ('P mitrale')
- Predominant negative component of P wave in V1

Right atrial enlargement

- P wave height of > 3 mm (tall 'P pulmonale')

Left bundle branch block (LBBB)

- QRS duration ≥ 0.12 s
- *and* absent initial Q wave in V5, V6, I and AVL (small Q in these leads is normal and results from septal depolarization by the left bundle of His)
- *and* no secondary R wave in V1 diagnostic of right bundle branch block (RBBB)

(In the presence of LBBB criteria for QRS, S-T and T wave normality do not apply and should not be commented on. In particular Q waves are not diagnostic of transmural myocardial infarction in the presence of LBBB. Abnormal left axis deviation is not a feature of LBBB.)

LBBB is always a sign of significant cardiac pathology (most often ischaemic heart disease or hypertension).

Right bundle branch block (RBBB)

- QRS duration ≥ 0.12 s
- *and* secondary R wave in V1

(In the presence of RBBB normal criteria for the QRS complex do apply, so pathological Q waves in this situation are diagnostic of infarction. Abnormal right axis deviation is not a feature of RBBB.)

RBBB can occur in otherwise normal hearts but usually accompanies pathology (again most frequently ischaemic heart disease or hypertension).

Left anterior hemiblock

(Block of the anterior fascicle of the left bundle while the posterior fascicle continues to conduct.)

- A mean frontal plane QRS axis more negative than −30°
- *and* absence of evidence of inferior myocardial infarction (i.e. no Q waves in leads II and AVF)

(In the presence of RBBB left anterior hemiblock implies that conduction to the ventricle depends solely on the posterior fascicle of the left bundle and may be tenuous.)

Left ventricular hypertrophy

There is no specific diagnostic feature. The diagnosis becomes more probable as more features are found to be present in a particular ECG.

Cumulative diagnostic features
- An R wave in V4–V6 of > 30 mm
- An S wave in V1–V3 of > 30 mm.
- Tallest R in V4–V6 plus deepest S in V1–V3 of > 40 mm
- R wave in AVL > 15 mm
- R wave in AVF > 20 mm
- Ventricular activation time longer than 0.04 s
- S-T depression in leads V4–V6, I and AVL (left-sided leads)
- T wave flattening or inversion in leads V4–V6, I and AVL

(Abnormal left axis deviation is *not* a feature.)

Right ventricular hypertrophy

- Dominant R wave in V1
- Abnormal right axis deviation (more positive than +90°)

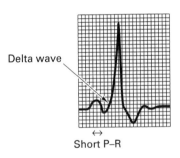

Delta wave

↔
Short P–R

Fig. 2.3

Wolff–Parkinson–White (WPW) syndrome   ventricular pre-excitation syndrome
⤷ WPW
⤷ LGL

- P-R interval of < 0.12 s
- *and* QRS duration > 0.12 s with slurring of the initial part of the QRS complex (delta wave)

(In the presence of WPW syndrome, criteria for QRS, S-T and T wave normality do not apply and should not be commented on. In the Lown–

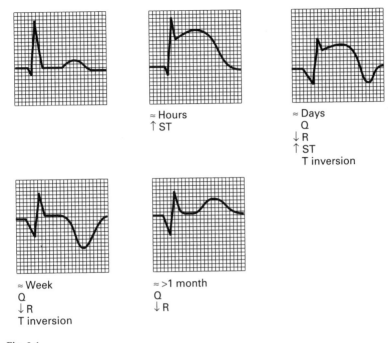

≈ Hours
↑ ST

≈ Days
Q
↓ R
↑ ST
T inversion

≈ Week
Q
↓ R
T inversion

≈ >1 month
Q
↓ R

Fig. 2.4

Ganong–Levine syndrome the P-R interval is short but there are no delta waves. Both syndromes are associated with bouts of paroxysmal tachycardia which can be very fast since the AV node is bypassed by the aberrant conducting pathway.)

Myocardial infarction

- Abnormal Q waves (see p. 150 for criteria of abnormality)
- Inappropriately low R waves in the chest leads (abnormal R wave progression)
- Observation of the sequence of ECG changes of infarction:
  1. Convex S-T elevation (usually persists a few days unless ventricular aneurysm develops when it may persist)
  2. Q waves
  3. T wave inversion
  4. Progressive ST and T wave normalization (T wave inversion persists for some weeks after ST segments have returned to normal)

Elevated serum cardiac enzymes support the diagnosis.

ECG changes indicative of myocardial infarction occur in characteristic leads depending on the site of the infarction:

Anterior infarction	V1–V6
Anterolateral infarction	V4–V6, I, AVL
Anteroseptal infarction	V1–V3
Inferior infarction	II, III, AVF
Inferolateral	II, III, AVF, V4–V6

Pericarditis

Generalized concave elevation of S-T segments (in all leads except those facing the ventricular cavity, i.e. always in AVR and also AVL when the heart is vertical and III when horizontal – cavity leads show S-T depression).

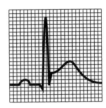

Fig. 2.5

Pulmonary embolism

Following acute pulmonary embolism the ECG is commonly normal. In cases of large embolism changes of acute right ventricular strain may be evident, including:

• Right axis deviation
• P pulmonale (increased P wave amplitude)
• RSR complex in lead V1
• Small Q waves in III and AVF
• Inverted T waves in V1–V3

Hyperkalaemia

Progressive changes with increasing potassium concentration:

1. Tall peaked T waves
2. Reduced P and R wave amplitude
3. Increased P-R interval
4. Widening of the QRS complex
5. Loss of isoelectric S-T segment

Complete heart block, ventricular tachycardia or ventricular fibrillation may occur in severe cases.

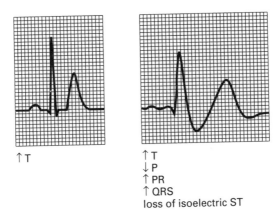

↑ T

↑ T
↓ P
↑ PR
↑ QRS
loss of isoelectric ST

Fig. 2.6

Hypokalaemia

Poor correlation of ECG changes with serum potassium concentration:

1. S-T segment depression
2. Reduced T wave amplitude
3. Increased U wave amplitude

Rarely, increased QRS duration or increased P wave amplitude.

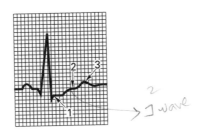

Fig. 2.7

Hypothermia

Bradycardia:

1. Prolonged P-R interval (first degree heart block)
2. A 'J' wave (characteristic secondary deflection towards the end of the QRS complex occurring at temperatures of 25°C or less)
3. Depressed S-T segments
4. T wave inversion

Atrial and ventricular fibrillation may occur.

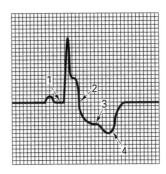

Fig. 2.8

Digoxin

ECG changes of digoxin are non-specific. They do not denote toxicity:

1. Decreased T wave amplitude
2. S-T segment depression (classically of 'reversed tick' configuration)
3. Increased U wave amplitude (usually slight)
4. shortening of the QT interval

Toxicity results in various dysrhythmias, including nodal and atrial tachycardias, ventricular ectopics (isolated or coupled), heart block, ventricular tachycardia, ventricular fibrillation.

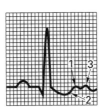

Fig. 2.9

ATRIAL DYSRHYTHMIAS

Sinus dysrhythmia

Some variation of rate of normal sinus rhythm (originating from the sino-atrial node) is usual in phase with respiration; the pulse rate increases during inspiration. Equally the rate of sinus rhythm varies in response to parasympathetic (vagal) and sympathetic influences.

When sinus rhythm is particularly slow 'escape' dysrhythmias are more likely; this simply means that abnormal rhythms can express themselves more easily when there is more time as when normal heart beats are not

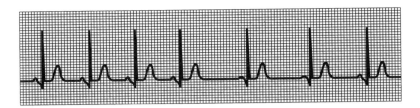

Fig. 2.10

occurring. In this situation increasing the heart rate with atropine may eradicate the dysrhythmia.

Nodal rhythm

When the sino-atrial node fails then the atrio-ventricular node will initiate depolarization, usually at a slower rate. His bundle conduction is normal so the QRS morphology is normal. There may be no P wave seen (Fig. 2.11a), or retrograde P wave conduction (Fig. 2.11b). When the rate is undesirably slow then it can be increased by atropine, which may also restore sinus rhythm. During anaesthesia discontinuation of halothane may have a similar effect.

(a)
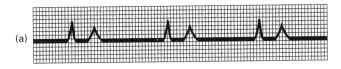

(b)
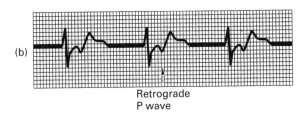
Retrograde
P wave

Fig. 2.11

Atrial ectopic beats (Fig. 2.12)

Discharges from an abnormal atrial focus may cause a premature depolarization. The P wave morphology may be abnormal or may be obscured by the previous T wave. The next beat follows at an interval which is frequently a little longer than the normal R-R interval.

Atrial ectopics usually require no treatment; where they are troublesome beta-blockers may eradicate them.

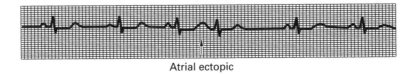

Atrial ectopic

Fig. 2.12

Supraventricular tachycardia

Denotes a tachydysrhythmia originating in the atrium or in the region of the atrio-ventricular node. The rate is characteristically 160–190/min and is usually short lived (paroxysmal). A rapidly discharging focus takes control of the heart rate. P waves may be clearly seen (Fig. 2.13a) which may differ from those seen in normal sinus rhythm in the same patient, but are often unclear (Fig. 2.13b).

When the ventricular rate is rapid, part of the His conducting system may prove inadequate and aberrant conduction may occur, resulting in widening of the QRS complexes (Fig. 2.13c); such cases are difficult to differentiate from ventricular tachycardia.

In supraventricular tachycardia the rhythm is absolutely regular without normal sinus dysrhythmia. Also, the clinical history does not reveal a clear cause to explain sinus tachycardia.

P wave
(superimposed on T waves)

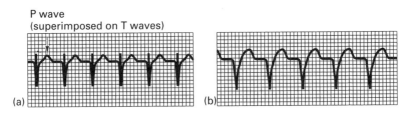

(a)   (b)

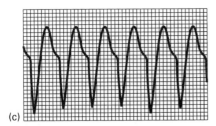

(c)

Fig. 2.13

Attacks may be curtailed by vagal influences (e.g. carotid sinus massage, edrophonium). Very rapid tachycardias with heart failure can be curtailed by synchronized DC cardioversion.

Drugs used in the treatment of supraventricular tachycardia include beta-blockers, verapamil (but beta-blockers and verapamil given simultaneously can result in heart block), flecainide.

Refractory cases may respond to amiodarone or radiofrequency ablation.

Atrial flutter

A specific, distinct type of supraventricular tachycardia with a very rapid atrial rate (characteristically 300/min). Classically there are clear, large, regular P waves termed 'F' (flutter) waves, which run into each other giving a 'saw-tooth' appearance particularly apparent in lead II. The rapid atrial rate exceeds that at which the atrio-ventricular node can conduct and a degree of heart block is inevitable resulting in an atrio-ventricular block.

Examples of atrial flutter with a 2:1 (Fig. 2.14a) or 4:1 (Fig. 2.14b) block are shown.

Reversion to sinus rhythm can be achieved by synchronized DC cardioversion.

The ventricular rate can be controlled by digoxin.

Atrial fibrillation

There is cessation of normal regular atrial depolarization, which is replaced by numerous random repolarizations of the atrium and incoordinate atrial

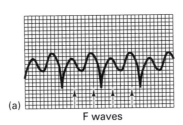
(a)
F waves

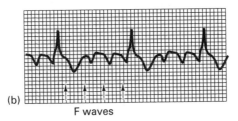
(b)
F waves

Fig. 2.14

action. Irregular undulation of the baseline of the ECG are usually apparent termed 'f' ('fibrillation') waves. Some impulses are transmitted randomly through the atrio-ventricular node. Such conduction may be rapid (up to 200/min) (Fig. 2.15a), resulting in heart failure, while slower rates of about 80/min (Fig. 2.15b) may be asymptomatic.

Acute cases can be restored to sinus rhythm by DC cardioversion.

In chronic cases the ventricular rate can be controlled by increasing the degree of atrio-ventricular block usually with digoxin but verapamil or beta-blockers can also be used.

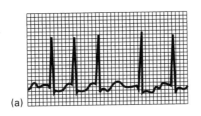

(a)

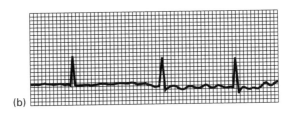

(b)

Fig. 2.15

VENTRICULAR DYSRHYTHMIAS

Ventricular ectopics

Ventricular ectopic beats result in widened QRS complexes, unrelated to a preceding P wave, occurring on a background of normal, narrow QRS complexes. The ectopic beat originates from an area of irritable myocardium and is not conducted through the His system and is therefore slower. Ectopics may be unifocal (all of identical morphology) (Fig. 2.16a) or multifocal (various different QRS morphologies of ectopic beats all of which are widened) (Fig. 2.16b).

Ventricular ectopic beats may occur in runs (Fig. 2.16c) or can precipitate ventricular tachycardia or ventricular fibrillation, particularly when the ectopic beat coincides with the T wave of the previous beat (Fig. 2.16d).

Ventricular ectopics usually require no treatment but may be treated with lidocaine (lignocaine). Other effective agents include mexiletine, flecainide, disopyramide and procainamide. Refractory cases may respond to amiodarone.

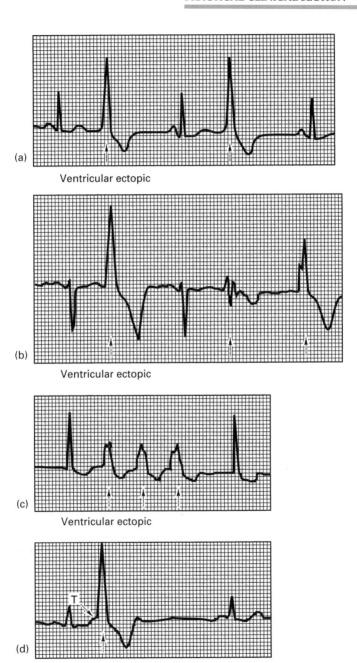

(a)

Ventricular ectopic

(b)

Ventricular ectopic

(c)

Ventricular ectopic

(d)

Fig. 2.16 Ventricular dysrhythmias.

Ventricular tachycardia

Repetitive discharge of an abnormal ventricular focus results in ventricular tachycardia. Ventricular tachycardia can revert spontaneously but may be sustained or degenerate to ventricular fibrillation.

During ventricular tachycardia cardiac output may be sustained, although unconsciousness is usual. The QRS complexes are broad and the rate rapid.

The rhythm in ventricular tachycardia may not be completely regular and the QRS morphology may not be uniform (Fig. 2.17a). However, differentiation from supraventricular tachycardia (with aberrant conduction) can be difficult (Fig. 2.17b).

Ventricular tachycardia is unresponsive to carotid sinus massage but is suppressed by the same drugs as are used for ventricular ectopics. Acute attacks of ventricular tachycardia usually require termination by synchronized DC cardioversion but drugs may prevent recurrent attacks.

HEART BLOCK

First-degree heart block

First-degree heart block is associated with a prolonged P-R interval (> 0.2 s) but no dropped beats (Fig. 2.18a). This form of heart block is common and does not generally progress to more serious forms.

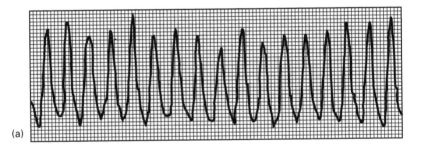

(a)

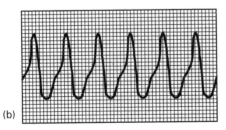

(b)

Fig. 2.17

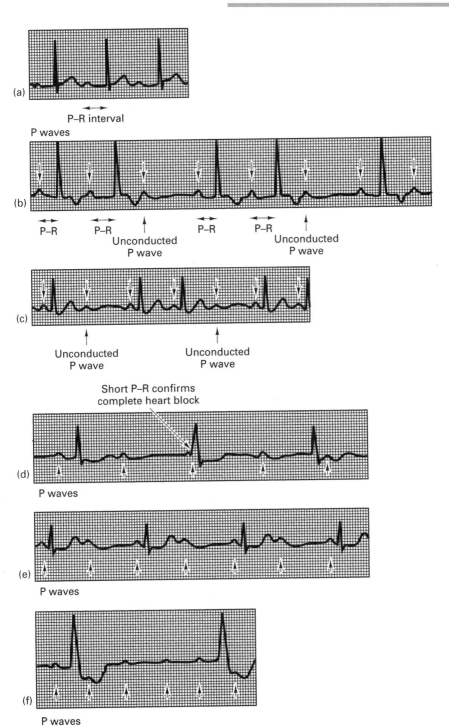

Fig. 2.18

Second-degree heart block

Second-degree heart block comprises two varieties, Wenckebach (Mobitz type I) and Mobitz type II.

- In Wenckebach heart block there is a progressive prolongation of the P-R interval and finally non-conduction of a P wave (Fig. 2.18b). There is then recovery of the atrio-ventricular node and the next P-R interval reverts to the previous shortest conduction time
- In Mobitz type II block there is a consistent P-R interval with intermittent non-conduction of some P waves (Fig. 2.18c)

In general, Wenckebach-type second-degree heart block is less likely to progress to complete heart block than is Mobitz type II heart block.

Complete heart block

Complete heart block (third-degree heart block) occurs when there is complete dissociation between the atrial and ventricular activity and each beats independently. There is no consistent relationship between the P wave and QRS complexes.

Sometimes it can be difficult to differentiate second-degree from third-degree block at first sight. When in doubt, short P-R intervals should be sought and this confirms complete block (the P wave is not intermittently conducting too quickly; the P wave and QRS complexes are independent and are almost occurring at the same time (Fig. 2.18d).

The ventricular rate in complete heart block depends on the site of ventricular pacemaker. A focus near the atrio-ventricular node produces regular complexes of narrow QRS configuration (since they are His conducted) at a rate of 50–60/min (Fig. 2.18e). (This is the situation in congenital complete heart block.) However, a low ventricular focus results in more irregular, wide QRS complexes at a rate of about 25–35/min (Fig. 2.18f). This rhythm is also unreliable and periods of asystole with syncope and possible death (the Stokes–Adams attack) are likely.

In heart block a slow ventricular rate may be increased by atropine or isoprenaline, usually as a temporary measure. Pervenous or endocardial demand pacing is more satisfactory and ensures against ventricular asystole.

Effects of anaesthesia

Anaesthesia may precipitate the development of complete heart block in susceptible cases due to reduction of A-V conduction by drugs (e.g. halothane) or alterations of K^+ concentration (suxamethonium, hypocapnia).

Indications for pacing wires to be inserted prior to anaesthesia

- In patients with fascicular block (especially LBBB) and a history of syncope (Stokes–Adams attack)

- In bifascicular block (RBBB and left anterior hemiblock) with delayed A-V conduction and a history of syncope
- Complete heart block (although pacing may not be required in cases with stable congenital heart block)
- Mobitz type II second-degree heart block (which is liable to progress to complete heart block)

Pacemaker code

Standardized pacemaker code to describe various types of pacemaker has been accepted:

Position I: The chamber paced
            V = Ventricle
            A = Atrium
            D = Both atrium and ventricle
            0 = None (antitachycardia but not for bradycardia
                pacing – rare)
Position II: The chamber sensed
            V = Ventricle
            A = Atrium
            D = Both atrium and ventricle
            0 = None
Position III: The response of the pacemaker to a sensed beat
            T = Triggered
            I = Inhibited (most common form of sensing)
            D = Double (atrium-triggered and ventricle-inhibited or
                both atrium- and ventricle-inhibited)
            0 = No response to sensed beat – totally committed pacing
                (asynchronous)
Position IV: Programmability, rate modulation
            P = Simple programmable (rate and/or output)
            M = Multiprogrammability
            C = Communicating (telemetry)
            R = Rate modulation (in response to patient activity or
                metabolic need)
            0 = None
Position V: Antitachycardia function
            P = Pacing (antitachycardia pacing)
            S = Shock
            D = Dual (pacing and shock available)
            0 = None

From a practical point of view, usually only the first three letters are used and an R is put at the end if rate modulation is an option.

Types of pacemaker (in common use)

VVI (ventricular demand pacemaker)

VVI is code for a single ventricular unipolar or bipolar wire attached to a pacemaker that paces in the ventricle and is inhibited by spontaneous electrical activation of the ventricle. In addition, many variables may be programmable, such as pulse rate, pulse width, refractory period, voltage output, sensitivity and hysteresis. This is by far the most common pacing mode used.

DDD

The DDD pacemaker is capable of sensing and pacing in both the atrium and ventricle. Virtually all dual-chamber pacemakers currently placed are DDDs. The DDD pacemaker is by far the most commonly used dual-chamber pacemaker. External programming of various parameters and modes of programming makes them highly versatile. The DDD mode functions as a rate-responsive pacemaker as long as the patient has adequate sinus mode or atrial rate that increases with exercise or stress. There is an upper rate beyond which atrial activity is not transmitted, to protect patients from atrial flutter/fibrillation.

In almost all pacemakers applying a magnet over the pacemaker generator will disable the sensing circuity so the pacemaker becomes asynchronous firing at a regular rate which ignores the patient's intrinsic activity.

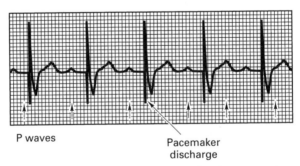

P waves   Pacemaker
discharge

- Sharp deflection preceding each QRS complex (due to pacemaker discharge)
- Prolonged QRS complex since depolarization begins at the periphery of the ventricle
- P waves may be observed, in which case they will bear no fixed relationship to the QRS complexes (where pacing performed as a result of complete heart block)

Fig. 2.19 Normal VVI rhythm.

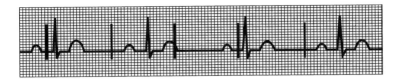

- The pacing spikes march through at a regular rate and are not inhibited by prior intrinsic electrical activity. Usually due to pacing wire displacement or fracture.

Fig. 2.20 Failure to capture or sense (VVI).

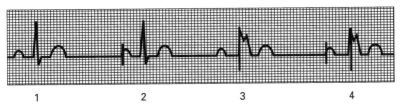

1. shows normal sinus rhythm
2. shows atrial pacing followed by normal AV conduction
3. shows normal atrial activity which is sensed by the pacemaker but not conducted and the ventricle is subsequently paced
4. shows both atrial and ventricular pacing

Fig. 2.21 DDD pacing.

X-RAYS

INTERPRETATION OF THE CHEST X-RAY

How to read a chest film

It is important to look at X-rays systematically. A system is suggested below but other systems are equally valid. It is important to assess X-rays swiftly in examinations, only mentioning positive observations and relative negative findings, particularly when there is an obvious lesion in the middle of the X-ray:

1. *Is it postero-anterior (P-A) or antero-posterior (A-P)?*
   A-P view magnifies the heart; generally signifies a sicker patient.
2. *Is it labelled (name, side)?*
   Name may signify racial origin and suggest particular diagnoses (e.g. tuberculosis).
3. *Is there any hardware?*
   Endotracheal tube, tracheostomy, central line, pulmonary arterial line, chest drain, pacemaker.

4. *Is the patient rotated or is there scoliosis?*
   This can alter radiographic density on the two sides of the chest.
5. *Is the penetration correct?*
   Posterior ribs should be just visible through the heart shadow.
   Do not criticize rotation and penetration unless gross: repeated technical criticism of each X-ray shown to a candidate can antagonize examiners.
6. *Are soft tissues normal?*
   Breasts – are both present? Lung base on side of mastectomy will be more radiolucent; possibility of secondaries suggested.
   Is there surgical emphysema?
7. *Is bony skeleton normal?*
   Systematically examine ribs, scapulae, humoral heads, clavicles and cervical spine. Particularly check for a cervical rib. Consider fractures, lytic lesions, degenerative disease and rib notching (indicative of aortic coarctation).
8. *Is the trachea central and inclining slightly to the right at the aortic knuckle?*
9. *Is the upper mediastinum of normal width?*
10. *Are the lung fields clear and of equal density? Are there signs of excess lung water? Do the peripheral vessels reach right to the chest wall?*
    Describe lesions as opacity which can be nodular, reticular, homogeneous, soft (fluffy) or well defined.
    If one lung field appears more dense than the other, establish whether this is abnormally dense or if the other is abnormally lucent (e.g. compensatory emphysema secondary to lobar collapse).
    If vessels are not clearly identifiable to the chest wall, look for the white line of lung edge of a pneumothorax, especially at the apex.
11. *Are the hila of normal outline and size and in the correct position? Are the fissures (if seen) in the correct position?*
12. *Is each dome of the diaphragm at the normal level? Are the costophrenic angles clear? Is there free gas under the diaphragm?*
13. *Is the heart of normal shape and outline?*
14. *Is the aortic shadow normal?*
    Double knuckle in coarctation.

SUMMARY

1. P-A or A-P?	9. Upper mediastinum
2. Labels	10. Lung fields
3. Hardware	11. Hila/fissures
4. Rotation/scoliosis	12. Diaphragm
5. Penetration	13. Heart
6. Soft tissues	14. Aorta
7. Bones	15. 'Hidden areas'
8. Trachea	

15. *Finally look carefully at the 'hidden areas':*
   — Behind and below the diaphragm
   — Behind the heart shadow
   — In the apices
   — The paratracheal region and upper mediastinum

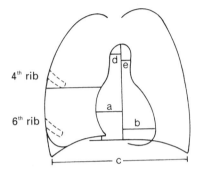
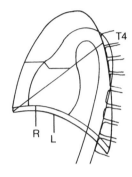

Fig. 2.22

Normal X-ray appearances

- There should be a good inspiration such that the right diaphragm lies below the level of the anterior end of the sixth rib
- The right diaphragm is 2.5 cm higher than the left. On the lateral view the right diaphragm should be clearly seen throughout its entire length, but the anterior part of the left is obscured due to its contact with the heart
- The lesser (horizontal) fissure lies at the level of the fifth thoracic vertebra posteriorly and at the level of the fourth rib anteriorly
- The greater (oblique) fissure is occasionally seen running inferomedially in the lateral part of the lower zone. On the lateral view the oblique fissure runs from T4 posteriorly to the diaphragm anteriorly
- The right hilum should be on the level of the lesser fissure, while the left is about 1 cm higher
- The cardiac shadow (on a P-A view) is less than half the thoracic diameter $(a + b < c/2)$
- The aortic shadow width is less than 4 cm $(d + e)$

DIFFERENTIAL DIAGNOSIS OF VARIOUS X-RAY APPEARANCES

- Unilateral hyperlucency
- Unilateral elevated diaphragm
- Widespread fine shadowing
- Nodular shadowing:

— Medium-sized nodules
— Single, large nodule
• Complete opacity of the hemithorax

Unilateral hyperlucency

• Rotation of the film
• Soft tissues (mastectomy, absent pectoralis)
• Increased density other side causing normal side to appear lucent
• Bullous cyst or cysts
• Pneumothorax
• Ball valve effect causing localized emphysema (most apparent on expiration)
• Compensatory emphysema secondary to lobar collapse or resection

Unilateral elevated diaphragm

• LMN phrenic palsy (no movement on quiet breathing, paradoxical elevation on sniffing)
• UMN phrenic palsy (poor movement on quiet breathing, no paradox on sniffing)
• Pulmonary collapse (when gross)
• Pulmonary infarct
• Scoliosis
• Space occupation below the diaphragm: .
— Subphrenic abscess
— Hepatic enlargement
— Ovarian cyst, etc.

Widespread fine shadowing

• Miliary tuberculosis
• Pulmonary oedema (including adult respiratory distress syndrome (ARDS))
• Infection – bronchopneumonia
• Pneumoconiosis/asbestosis
• Dust inhalation (talc, cadmium, barium)
• Fibrosing alveolitis (Hamman–Rich)
• Sarcoidosis
• Allergic alveolitis
• Lymphangitis carcinomatosis
• ARDS
• Following lymphangiogram

Nodular shadowing

Medium-sized nodules
• Infection

- Tuberculosis
- Secondary neoplasia
- Rheumatoid (Caplan's syndrome where pneumoconiosis-associated)

Single large nodule
- Bronchogenic carcinoma
- Secondary neoplasia
- Adenoma/hamartoma
- Abscess
- Arteriovenous malformation
- Aspergilloma
- Tuberculosis
- Encysted pleural fluid

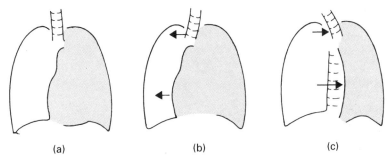

(a)   (b)   (c)

a. Total unilateral lung consolidation
- Homogeneous opacity
- Loss of outlines of cardiac border and hemidiaphragm
- Mediastinum not displaced
- Trachea central

b. Massive pleural effusion
- Homogeneous opacity
- Loss of outlines of cardiac border and hemidiaphragm
- Mediastinum displaced away from side of opacity
- Trachea displaced away from side of opacity

c. Total unilateral lung collapse or pneumonectomy
- Homogeneous opacity
- Loss of outlines of cardiac border and hemidiaphragm
- Loss of outlines of cardiac border and hemidiaphragm
- Mediastinum displaced towards side of opacity (cardiac border may be obscured over vertebrac which may come into view)
- Trachea displaced towards side of opacity
- Signs of rib resection may suggest pneumonectomy and lung secondaries may be present. An air fluid level at the top of the opacity suggests bronchopleural fistula
- Diaphragm raised

Fig. 2.23

SPECIFIC X-RAY APPEARANCES

- Consolidation
- Collapse
- Pleural effusion
- Pleural effusion with pneumothorax
- Pneumothorax
- Emphysema
- Cystic fibrosis
- Achalasia of the oesophagus
- Bronchiectasis
- Lung abscess
- Hiatus hernia
- Superior mediastinal swelling
- Coarctation of the aorta
- Pulmonary oedema
- Mitral stenosis
- Eisenmenger's syndrome
- Fallot's tetralogy
- Pericardial effusion
- Cervical spine:
  — Ankylosing spondylitis
  — Rheumatoid arthritis
  — Severe osteoarthritis
  — Klippel–Feil syndrome
  — Fracture dislocation

Consolidation

- Usually homogeneous area of increased shadowing
- Bounded by a segmental margin
- When marked may produce an air bronchogram
- Often associated with a degree of collapse
- Exhibits the 'silhouette sign'

The 'silhouette sign' results from localized loss of normal margins. Recognition of this sign aids localization of areas of consolidation.

Loss of silhouette (Fig. 2.24)
1. Lateral segment middle lobe
2. Medial segment middle lobe
3. Anterior segment lower lobe
4. Lateral segment lower lobe
5. Anterior segment upper lobe
6. Apicoposterior segment upper lobe
7. Lingula

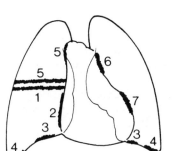

Fig. 2.24

Retained silhouette (Fig. 2.25)
1. Posterior segment lower lobe
2. Dorsal segment lower lobe
3. Posterior segment upper lobe
4. Anterior segment upper lobe

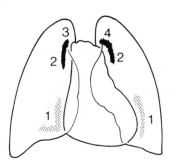

Fig. 2.25

Collapse

- Segmental area of increased density (only when there is virtual complete collapse or some associated consolidation)
- Loss of lung volume:
  — Displacement of fissure towards collapsed lobe
  — Rotary displacement of the pulmonary artery towards collapse
  — Displacement of the diaphragm and mediastinum towards collapse (only with large areas of collapse)
- Compensatory emphysema and scarcity of vessels in remaining lung

Right upper lobe (Fig. 2.26)
1. Elevation of the lesser fissure on A-P view and displacement of both greater and lesser fissures on lateral view
2. Right paratracheal shadow with crowding of vessels within collapsing lobe
3. Compensatory emphysema in remaining lung
4. Rotary elevation of the pulmonary artery. Diaphragm and mediastinum not usually displaced

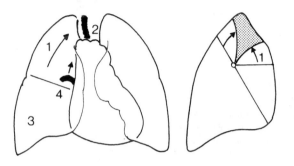

Fig. 2.26

Right middle lobe (Fig. 2.27)
1. Depression of the lesser fissure (often invisible on the A-P view)
2. Silhouette sign right cardiac border

Pulmonary artery, diaphragm and mediastinum not usually displaced. Small lobe so little compensatory emphysema in other lobes.

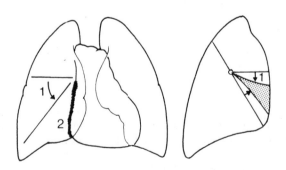

Fig. 2.27

Right lower lobe (Fig. 2.28)
1. Depression of the lesser fissure on A-P view. Greater fissure also displaced on lateral view (appears to pass well behind the hilum)

2. Area of density at or behind the right cardiac border
3. Depression of the pulmonary artery
4. Silhouette sign right diaphragm
5. Compensatory emphysema in remaining lung

Diaphragm or mediastinal displacement unusual.

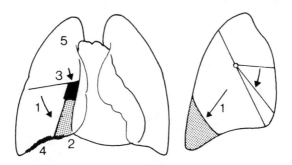

Fig. 2.28

Left upper lobe (Fig. 2.29)
1. Increased lung density in the region of the aortic knuckle
2. Silhouette sign at aortic knuckle and involvement of the lingula causes silhouette sign at left heart border
3. Greater fissure displaced on lateral view (appears to pass in front of hilum)
4. Substernal hyperlucent area (as normal aerated lung tissue moves round as upper lobe retracts)
5. Compensatory emphysema in remaining lung

Pulmonary artery, diaphragm and mediastinum not usually displaced.

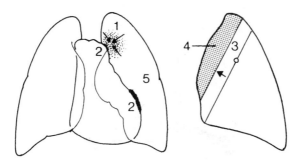

Fig. 2.29

Left lower lobe (Fig. 2.30)
1. Increased density retracting behind the heart
2. Displacement of the greater fissure on the lateral view
3. Depression of the pulmonary artery
4. Silhouette sign on left diaphragm
5. Compensatory emphysema in remaining lung

Diaphragm and mediastinum not usually displaced.

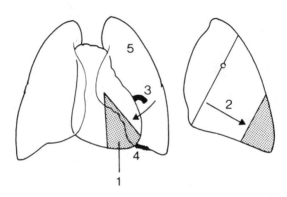

Fig. 2.30

Pleural effusion (Fig. 2.31)

- Homogenous basal opacity in effect film starting in the costophrenic angle
- Curved upper margin – forms when reaches >200–300 ml
- Changes with posture (unless loculated); becomes a diffuse haze through which lung markings can be seen when patient is supine – therefore bilateral effusions easily missed

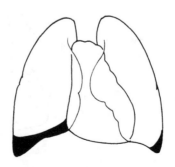

Fig. 2.31

Pleural effusion with pneumothorax (Fig. 2.32)

• Fluid in the pleural space with air above gives a straight superior
  margin

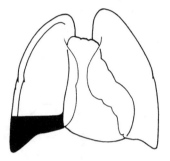

Fig. 2.32

Pneumothorax (Fig. 2.33)

• Air in the pleural space with relaxation of the lung
• More relaxation evident on expiration film
• A thin white line of the lung margin with no lung markings beyond
• Where tension pneumothorax is present the mediastinum and
  diaphragm are displaced away from the side of the tension
• Beware small apical pneumothorax on otherwise normal film
• Look for a cause – e.g. rib fractures, central venous line

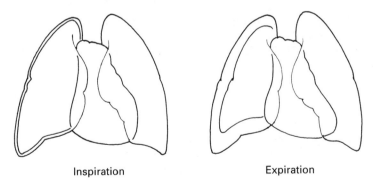

Inspiration   Expiration

Fig. 2.33

Supine pneumothorax (Fig. 2.34)
When the patient is supine pleural air rises and the lung falls to the posterior part of the thorax so no lung edge may be seen.

Signs which suggest pneumothorax include:

1. Generalized translucency of a hemithorax which may extend into and deepen the costophrenic angle
2. Depression of the hemidiaphragm
3. Visualization of the undersurface of the heart
4. A band-like translucency parallel to the diaphragm and or mediastinum with undue clarity of the mediastinal border

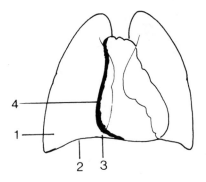

Fig. 2.34

Diagnosis of pneumothorax in the supine patient is assisted by:

- Taking an erect picture (often not possible in sick patients)
- Taking a lateral decubitus film
- Performing a CT slice through the thorax (particularly when the patient requires imaging of other regions)

Emphysema (Fig. 2.35)

1. Flat diaphragms
2. Diaphragms below the anterior end of the seventh rib
3. Gap between the left diaphragm and the cardiac border
4. Barrel chest with posterior ribs lying horizontally
5. Small heart shadow
6. Coarse lung marking due to sputum accumulation in airways and mucous gland hypertrophy where chronic bronchitis is associated
7. Bullae may be present

Increased anterior mediastinal air space and increased A-P chest diameter on lateral view.

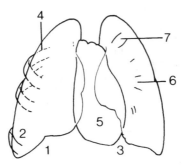

Fig. 2.35

Cystic fibrosis (Fig. 2.36)

1. Hyperinflation (as emphysema)
2. Diffuse reticular shadowing
3. Cystic change of honeycombing in advanced cases
4. Prominent bronchi due to mucosal hypertrophy
5. 'Gloved finger' of bronchiectasis (mucus-filled dependent bronchi)
6. Prominent pulmonary artery where pulmonary hypertension has developed
7. Young appearance of bones. (Prognosis is poor so patients tend to be young. The X-ray looks like that of a 90-year-old, while the bones are those of an adolescent.)

Achalasia of the oesophagus (Fig. 2.37)

1. Dilated oesophagus, often with a fluid level
2. Possible associated evidence of aspiration with consolidation abscess formation or fibrosis. Especially of the dorsal segment of the right lower lobe due to regurgitation at night while supine

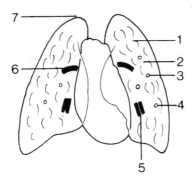

Fig. 2.36

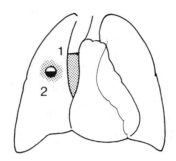

Fig. 2.37

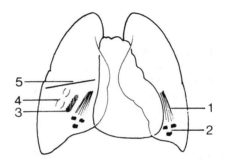

Fig. 2.38

Bronchiectasis (Fig. 2.38)

1. Increased lung markings, especially along cardiac borders
2. Scattered patchy consolidation
3. Visualization of dilated, mucus-filled bronchi
4. Visualization of thickened walls of dilated bronchi
5. Frequent associated collapse

Lung abscess (Fig. 2.39)

1. Abscess cavity with fluid level
2. Usually originates from an area of consolidation
3. Usually some associated collapse (evidenced by a depressed lesser fissure in this example)

Hiatus hernia (Fig. 2.40)

An air fluid level behind the heart, which may project from the left cardiac border (and also rarely from the right border).

Diagnosis can be supported by a lateral view and established on barium swallow.

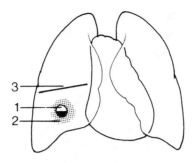

Fig. 2.39

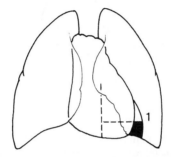

Fig. 2.40

Superior mediastinal swelling (Fig. 2.41)

Important causes include retrosternal goitre and thymic tumour. A lateral X-ray is very important to localize the site of the mass:

1. Widening of the upper mediastinum
2. Deviation distortion and possible narrowing of the trachea

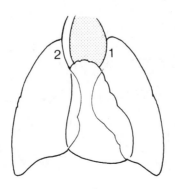

Fig. 2.41

Coarctation of the aorta (Fig. 2.42)

1. Double small aortic knuckle
2. Rib notching (takes some years to become evident)
3. Usually young patient's X-rays shown

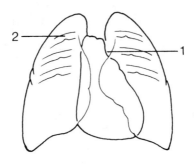

Fig. 2.42

Pulmonary oedema (Fig. 2.43)

1. Distended upper lobe veins
2. Kerley B septal lines (short horizontal lines at the periphery of the lower zone)
3. Kerley A septal lines (long fine lines in the upper zone radiating from the hilum)
4. Diffuse hazy shadowing radiating from the hilar region, mostly above the fissure and in the lower zone. Blurring of the hilum. Shadowing may appear blotchy and nodular. ('Bat's wing' distribution is characteristic.)
5. Pleural effusions (usually small)
6. Cardiac enlargement (or failure)

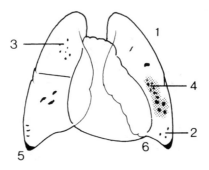

Fig. 2.43

Mitral stenosis (Fig. 2.44)

Signs of high pulmonary venous pressure
1. Kerley B septal lines
2. Kerley A septal lines
3. Prominent lesser fissure due to interfissural fluid
4. Prominent upper lobe veins (upper lobe diversion)
5. Pulmonary oedema; dilated left atrium
6. Straight left heart border (enlarged left atrial appendage)
7. Double shadow right cardiac border
8. Elevation of the left main bronchus (lateral barium swallow may also show dilated atrium)

Other features
9. Calcification of the mitral valve (sometimes of the left atrium also)
10. Dilated pulmonary arteries secondary to pulmonary hypertension in advanced cases
11. Normal heart size usual in uncomplicated cases

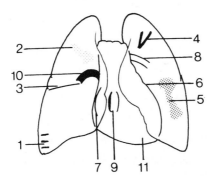

Fig. 2.44

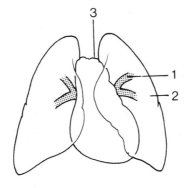

Fig. 2.45

Eisenmenger's syndrome (Fig. 2.45)

Reversal of a left-to-right shunt as a result of pulmonary hypertension:

1. Large dilated main pulmonary arteries
2. Oligaemia of peripheral lung fields
3. Small aortic shadow (resulting from long-standing left-to-right shunt)

Fallot's tetralogy (Fig. 2.46)

1. Apex of heart raised above level of hemidiaphragm
2. Pulmonary oligaemia with small pulmonary arteries
3. Dilated aorta

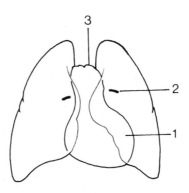

Fig. 2.46

Pericardial effusion (Fig. 2.47)

1. Large globular cardiac shadow; rather symmetrical enlargement both sides of the midline
2. Clear heart border (since cardiac movement is obscured by fluid – normally cardiac movement causes some blurring especially with tachycardia)
3. Absent signs of heart failure

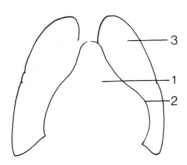

Fig. 2.47

Cervical spine

Important conditions with anaesthetic significance (and which are liable to feature in examinations) include:

Ankylosing spondylitis
- Loss of anterior concavity of vertebrae (vertebrae becoming squared)
- Calcification of paraspinal ligaments (resulting in the 'bamboo spine' appearance)
- Loss of normal cervical lordosis and loss of movement
- Restricted cervical spine movement results in difficult intubation

Rheumatoid arthritis
- Erosions, osteoporosis, subluxations and secondary osteoarthritic changes (osteophytes)
- Subluxation can occur at any cervical level but is particularly at the C1/C2 level (atlanto-axial subluxation). It is demonstrated by flexion–extension views. On the flexion view the distance from the posterior part of the anterior arch of the atlas to the anterior part of the odontoid process should be less than 4 mm in patients younger than 44 years, and less than 3 mm in older patients
- Limitation of cervical spine movement and temporomandibular joint ankylosis (secondary to rheumatoid involvement) can make intubation difficult. Cases of myelopathy due to subluxation can be exacerbated (possible to the extent of producing quadriplegia) by cervical spine movement during attempted intubation or positioning for surgery

Severe osteoarthritis (spondylosis)
- Marked osteophyte formation and osteosclerosis
- A reasonable range of cervical spine movement is usual. Osteophytic encroachment of intervertebral foramina results in irritation of nerve roots. Rotation of the head may cause temporary brain stem ischaemia when atheroma is associated; care in positioning such patients for surgery is important

Klippel–Feil syndrome
Developmental malformation due to defective segmentation of cervical vertebrae (rarely, thoracic or lumbar levels can be involved):

- Fusion of cervical vertebrae (both bodies and neural arch can be fused). Results in a short neck with limited mobility (especially rotation)
- Associated with spina bifida and cervical rib
- Short, immobile neck is likely to be associated with severe intubation difficulties

Fracture dislocation
- Loss of normal curvature of cervical spine with a 'step' and prevertebral swelling. Vertebrae may be compressed or there may be avulsed fragments; fractures of the neural arch may also be seen

- Movement of an unstable cervical spine (including that movement required for direct laryngoscopy) is undesirable as further cord damage may result

Other considerations

Where cervical spine X-rays do not appear to show any of the above conditions consider whether the mandible is hypoplastic (indicating that intubation may be difficult) and look at the larynx (there may be a foreign body or globular enlargement of the epiglottis and/or aryepiglottic folds characteristic of epiglottitis).

INTRACRANIAL HAEMATOMAS

Extradural haematomas

Acute extradural haematoma is usually due to arterial bleeding from the middle meningeal artery; plain skull films frequently show a fracture crossing the groove of that vessel in the temporoparietal region.

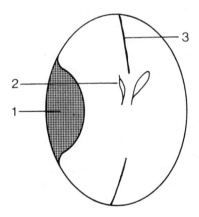

Fig. 2.48

1. Haematoma assumes an ellipsoid shape with a biconvex lentiform high density area immediately underlying the vault
2. Contralateral displacement of the brain with ventricular compression
3. Midline shift

Subdural haematomas

Acute subdural haematoma is usually associated with damage to the brain and arises mainly from rupture of veins in the subdural space. Subacute subdural collections, presenting 7–10 days after injury are less commonly accompanied by fractures than in acute cases:

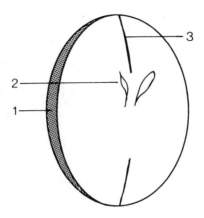

Fig. 2.49

1. Haematoma assumes a more or less crescentic or concavoconvex lens appearance. This is because the blood within it is under less pressure, but is less restricted in extent
2. Contralateral displacement of the brain with ventricular compression
3. Midline shift

Highly proteinaceous blood components cause high radiographic density, distinguishing clot from adjacent brain. After a few days, the density of the clot begins to decrease and it will pass through a period when it is the same density as brain. After 2 or more weeks, the clot is less dense than brain.

PULMONARY FUNCTION TESTS

Questions covering these tests are frequently seen in the multiple choice examination and in the clinical viva. A clear understanding of these various tests is essential to the examination candidate. Below is a list of respiratory and ventilatory parameters (and their abbreviations) that may occur.

Respiratory and ventilatory parameters

- Total lung capacity (TLC)
- Vital capacity (VC)
- Inspiratory capacity (IC)
- Functional residual capacity (FRC)
- Tidal volume (V_T)
- Inspiratory reserve volume (IRV)

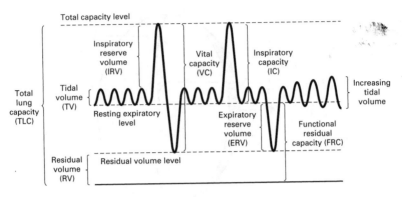

Fig. 2.50

- Expiratory reserve volume (ERV)
- Residual volume (RV)
- Dead space (V_D)
- Alveolar ventilation ($\overset{\circ}{V}_A$)
- Forced expiratory volume in 1 s (FEV_1)
- Forced vital capacity (FVC)
- Peak expiratory flow rate (PEFR)
- Maximum breathing capacity (MBC)

Some of these parameters may be measured by the use of a simple spirometer in the ward, others require the more sophisticated equipment available in a pulmonary function laboratory. These tests should be reviewed prior to the examination. The commonest tests seen in clinical practice and in examinations are spirometric and are dealt with below.

Spirometric tests

If a patient exhales as fast and for as long as possible from full inspiration into a spirometer, the volume expired in the first second is the FEV_1 and the total expired is the FVC (Fig. 2.51a).

Constriction of major airways (e.g. in asthma) reduces the FEV_1 more than the FVC. This results in a FEV_1/FVC ratio less than the normal of 0.7 (Fig. 2.51b).

Restriction of the lungs (e.g. in fibrosis) reduces the FVC and, to a lesser extent, the FEV_1. This results in a FEV_1/FVC ratio of 0.7 or greater (Fig. 2.51c).

The shape of the curve produced by the spirometer should be inspected and used with the result of the above simple calculations when assessing a patient's respiratory function.

The PEFR is a measure of the maximum rate of flow of exhaled air during a forced expiration. In practice it provides similar information to the FEV_1 and is a measure of obstructive disease.

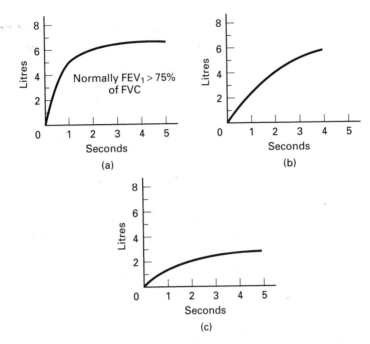

Fig. 2.51

The maximum breathing capacity (MBC) is measured by ensuring the subject breathes as deeply and as fast as he/she can for 15 s and measuring the volume of exhaled air. This measurement also correlates well with the FEV_1 but is much more distressing to the subject and depends far more on his/her cooperation.

The tests are frequently repeated following the administration of a beta$_2$ sympathomimetic agent such as salbutamol, thus allowing an assessment of the degree of reversibility of any obstructive component.

BLOOD GAS ANALYSIS

Normal values

Normal values are given in Table 2.1.

Definitions of values

pH
Negative logarithm of the relative activity of hydrogen ions in the blood plasma (alternatively the actual hydrogen concentration (SI unit) in nmol/l

Table 2.1 Normal blood gas values

pH	7.34–7.44 (45.7–36.3 nmol/l)
P_{CO_2}	4.4–5.8 kPa (33–43 mmHg)
P_{O_2}	10.0–13.3 kPa (80–110 mmHg)
Hb	12.5–17.0 g/100 ml
T_{CO_2}	22–32 mmol/l
HCO_3	20–30 mmol/l
SBC	20–30 mmol/l
ABE and SBE	−2.5–2.5 mmol/l
SAT	95–98%
O_2CT	15–23 vol%

is quoted). The result will be more basic if the analysis is made at a lower temperature than that of the patient. Conversely when the patient is cold during hypothermia the result of an analysis at 37°C will be more acidic.

The importance of correction for temperature is unclear; however, if correction is made, then a factor of −0.0147 unit of pH per degree centigrade is used: thus for a patient at 27°C the normal pH when measured at 37°C will be 7.25 (7.4 − 0.147 = 7.25).

P_{CO_2} and P_{O_2}

The partial pressure of each in the gas phase in equilibrium with the blood.

Hb

Haemoglobin concentration determined photometrically according to Beer's law.

T_{CO_2} (total CO_2)

Concentration of CO_2, both free and bound, in the plasma. Also has both respiratory and metabolic components:

$$T_{CO_2} = HCO_3 + (P_{CO_2} \times solubility)$$

HCO_3

Concentration of bicarbonate in plasma calculated from the pH and P_{CO_2} using the Henderson–Hasselbalch equation:

$$pH = pKa + log(HCO_3/P_{CO_2})$$

The Siggard–Andersen formula is used to give a linear relationship between pH and pK. Metabolic and respiratory components contribute to the bicarbonate result.

SBC (standard bicarbonate concentration)

Concentration of bicarbonate in the plasma from blood which is equilibrated with a gas with P_{CO_2} of 5.32 kPa (40 mmHg). This is thus a measure of 'metabolic' bicarbonate, since the P_{CO_2} is controlled.

ABE (actual base excess)

The difference in concentration of strong base in whole blood and in the same blood titrated with strong acid or base to pH 7.4 at P_{CO_2} of 5.32 kPa (40 mmHg) and 37°C. It is calculated from an empirical formula describing the Siggard–Andersen curve nomogram. Since P_{CO_2} is controlled, this is a measure of metabolic alkalosis (or acidosis). Negative results indicate metabolic acidosis.

SBE (standard base excess)

The ABE is an in vitro expression of metabolic imbalance. In vivo the buffering capacity of interstitial fluid is lower than that of whole blood (since there is no haemoglobin and lower protein in interstitial fluid). The ABE is therefore adjusted to give a measure of in vivo buffering, the SBE.

SAT (oxygen saturation)

The amount of O_2 which is combined with haemoglobin, divided by the amount of O_2 which can be combined with haemoglobin (i.e. content/capacity).

O_2CT (oxygen content)

The concentration of O_2 in the blood including both oxyhaemoglobin and dissolved haemoglobin.

Simple scheme for interpretation of blood gases

1. Look at the pH and determine acidosis or alkalosis
2. Look at the P_{CO_2} and standard bicarbonate to determine respiratory and metabolic components: the primary abnormality (respiratory or metabolic) is always that which explains the observed pH.
   Compensation is almost always incomplete and only moderates the effect of the primary abnormality
3. Look at the haemoglobin
4. Look at the P_{O_2} (and the F_iO_2 where marked)

Compensation limits

See Table 2.2.

Some patterns of abnormality

The arterial blood gas results in Table 2.3 illustrate some patterns of abnormality.

Example 1
Mild acidosis with respiratory and metabolic components.

Example 2
Acidosis which is metabolic. The P_{CO_2} is low indicating compensatory respiratory alkalosis which moderates the effect of the metabolic deficit on pH. This is the picture of diabetic ketoacidosis.

Table 2.2 Compensation limits

Disorder	Primary lesion	Compensation	Compensation limits
Metabolic acidosis	$\downarrow[HCO_3^-]$	$\downarrow Pco_2$	Limit: Pco_2~1–2 kPa Expected Pco_2 mmHg: $0.75 \times [HCO_3^-] + 8 \pm 2$
Metabolic alkalosis	$\uparrow[HCO_3^-]$	$\uparrow Pco_2$	Limit: Pco_2~55–60 mmHg Expected Pco_2 mmHg: $0.9 \times [HCO_3^-] + 9$
Respiratory acidosis			
Acute	$\uparrow Pco_2$	$\uparrow[HCO_3^-]$	Limit: $[HCO_3^-]$~30 mmol/l Expected $[HCO_3^-]$ mmol: $\uparrow$by 2–4
Chronic	$\uparrow Pco_2$	$\uparrow[HCO_3^-]$	Limit: $[HCO_3^-]$~44 mmol/l Expected $[HCO_3^-]$ mmol: $0.36 \times Pco_2 + 10$
Respiratory alkalosis			
Acute	$\downarrow Pco_2$	$\downarrow[HCO_3^-]$	Limit: $[HCO_3^-]$~18 mmol Expected $[HCO_3^-]$ mmol/l: $\downarrow$by 2–4
Chronic	$\downarrow Pco_2$	$\downarrow[HCO_3^-]$	Limit: $[HCO_3^-]$~12 mmol/l Expected: pH to~7.40

Table 2.3 Examples of abnormalities

	(1)	(2)	(3)	(4)	(5)
Hb	13.2	13.2	9.7	18.2	8.0 g/100 ml
pH	7.289	7.081	7.532	7.275	7.46
Pco_2	6.02	2.76	3.83	12.98	2.59 kPa
Po_2	10.13	14.10	4.44	4.44	13.49 kPa
HCO_3	21.1	5.9	23.7	44.0	13.8 mmol/l
Tco_2	22.4	6.5	24.5	47.0	14.4 mmol/l
ABE	−5.2	−23.5	2.0	11.4	−8.9 mmol/l
SBE	−4.7	−22.4	1.4	15.8	−9.3 mmol/l
SBC	19.9	8.4	25.7	33.9	17.2 mmol/l
SAT	91.9	94.9	67.2	55.1	98.0%
O_2CT	19.9	17.7	9.2	13.9	11.2 vol%

Example 3
Alkalosis which is respiratory in origin. Lack of metabolic compensation suggests acute onset. Low Po_2. This is the picture of hypoxic drive (e.g. due to an acute chest infection).

Example 4

Mild acidosis which is respiratory. There is a high bicarbonate and base excess (SBE) indicating a compensatory metabolic alkalosis. There is also a high haemoglobin and hypoxia. This is the picture of chronic respiratory failure.

Example 5

Alkalosis which is respiratory in origin. However, note metabolic acidosis also present, which is larger than one would expect in compensation. This picture is of aspirin overdose which causes a metabolic acidosis plus a respiratory alkalosis by direct stimulation of the respiratory centre. Note also low haemoglobin.

ELECTROLYTE INTERPRETATION

HYPONATRAEMIA

Causes

- Pseudohyponatraemia
- Hypertonic hyponatraemia
- Hypotonic hyponatraemia

Pseudohyponatraemia

Only seen when sodium is measured by an 'indirect reading' electrode or flame photometer (the usual method in biochemistry laboratories) but not when measured by a direct reading electrode (the usual method in combined blood gas and electrolyte analysers).

93% normal plasma is water. Increased lipid or protein will decrease the percentage water.

- Triglyceride > 5 mmol/l or total protein > 150 gm/l will influence indirect results

(measured osmol = OK, osmolar gap will be present)

Hypertonic hyponatraemia

Plasma, hyperglycaemia, mannitol.

Water movement from intracellular to extracellular space resulting in dilution of plasma contents (unusual since hyperglycaemia and mannitol usually cause an osmotic diuresis which causes a greater loss of plasma water and consequently hypernatraemia).

In hyperglycaemia dividing the glucose by 4 and adding this to the measured plasma sodium will give a 'true' plasma sodium (i.e. the sodium concentration which would be present if the excess glucose and water were removed from the extracellular fluid).

Hypotonic hyponatraemia

Usual type of hyponatraemia due to a positive water balance.

The inability to excrete a dilute urine in the presence of hypotonicity may be due to:

- Decreased delivery of fluid to the renal diluting segments, e.g. hypovolaemia causing an increased proximal tubular reabsorption of salt and water
- Defective function of the diluting segment (ascending limb of loop of Henle), e.g. loop diuretics such as furosemide (frusemide), renal disease
- Continued secretion of ADH despite hypotonicity of the extracellular fluid:
  — Hypovolaemia
  — Stress
  — Drugs
    Increased ADH secretion
    – morphine
    – chlorpropamide
    – carbamazepine
    – vincristine, vinblastine
    Potentiation of ADH action
    – chlorpropamide
    – indomethacin
    Diuretics
  — SIADH (syndrome of inappropriate secretion of ADH)

Effects
Depend on rapidity of change in acute situation: a sodium level < 125 mmol/l is usually symptomatic – chronic cases may be asymptomatic at sodium levels above 115 mmol/l.

Clinical features includes nausea, malaise, muscle weakness, delirium, coma and seizures.

Treatment
Treatment is controversial.

In acute cases (hours only) relatively rapid increase of plasma sodium to 125 mmol/l is probably generally acceptable. Thereafter slower increase to normal values is appropriate since 125 mmol/l is a safe level.

In chronic treatment depends on symptoms. Patients with few symptoms do not require rapid restoration and such aggressive treatment may be associated with severe subsequent neurological deficit (central pontine myelinolysis). Severe cases presenting with convulsions and depressed consciousness should be treated in a similar fashion to acute cases (see above).

HYPERNATRAEMIA

Results in intracellular dehydration lethargy, coma, muscle weakness, thirst, but when chronic there is an increase in intracellular osmolality ('idiogenic osmoles') which compensates for the extracellular hyperosmolality. Rapid restoration of chronic hypernatraemia to normal is not therefore indicated and may lead to the development of cerebral oedema.

Causes

- Water depletion – inadequate intake, increased loss (fever, etc.), diabetes insipidus
- Hypotonic fluid loss (mixed isotonic fluid loss and water loss)
- GI (vomiting, diarrhoea), renal (osmotic diuresis)
- Salt gain – hypertonic sodium bicarbonate, sodium chloride administration
- More likely in the very young and the very old

POTASSIUM

Major intracellular cation. 80 mmol extracellular, 4400 mmol intracellular.

Hyperkalaemia

Causes
- Factitious increase in K^+ (haemolysis at or after blood collection)
- Increased overall body K^+ status
- Shift of K^+ out of cells
  — Cell death and lysis (e.g. haemolysis, rhabdomyolysis, suxamethonium use in burns or spinal patients)
  — Cellular acidosis (cellular H^+ accumulation in acidosis results in extracellular K^+ movement to maintain cellular electrical neutrality)

Effects
Increased $K^+ > 4.5$ mmol/l, muscle weakness, flaccid paralysis and paraesthesiae. Cardiac arrhythmia and ECG change.

- Peaked T waves (6–7 mmol/l)
- Aberrant QRS complexes (8–10 mmol/l)
- Fused QRS and T waves (11 mmol/l)
- VT (10–12 mmol/l)

Treatment
Since factitious increased K^+ is common always repeat sample and ECG monitor patient before initiating aggressive treatment.

- Calcium gluconate (transient antagonism of cardiac effect of increased K^+)
- Sodium bicarbonate. Effect lasts for some hours
- Glucose and insulin. Effect lasts for some hours
- Resonium A (sodium polystyrene sulphonate) exchanges Na^+ for K^+ in the gut
- Haemofiltration

Hypokalaemia

Causes
- Factitious low K (drip arm blood sampling)
- Decreased overall body K^+ status
  — Renal aldosterone = K^+ loss + Na^+ retention – spironolactone antagonizes
  — Distal renal tubular flow (e.g. diuretic) increased flow = increased K^+ loss
  — Alkalosis = increased K^+ in renal tubular cells with bigger gradient = K^+ loss
  — Diarrhoea, vomit (up to 100 mmol/l K^+ in diarrhoea)
- Shift of K^+ into cells
  — Insulin increases cellular K^+ uptake
  — Adrenaline (epinephrine) increases cellular K^+ uptake by beta-receptor stimulation

Effects
$K^+ < 3.5$ mmol/l.

Anorexia, nausea, polyuria (nephrogenic diabetes insipidus of hypokalaemia) muscle weakness, paralysis.

Treatment
- Elimination of cause of loss where possible
- Increased potassium intake (not more than 2 g/h unless monitored)

ANION GAP ACIDOSIS

Anion gap = 'unmeasured anions'.

Anion gap = $(Na + K) - (Cl + HCO_3^-)$.

Metabolic acidosis (reduction of bicarbonate) must be associated with either an increase of the anion gap (anion gap acidosis) or of the chloride (non-anion gap or hyperchloraemic acidosis) since the overall quantity of cations and anions must match.

Bicarbonate loss from the gut or kidney with replacement by chloride-containing fluid will result in a non-anion gap or hyperchloraemic acidosis.

Causes of an increased anion gap include:

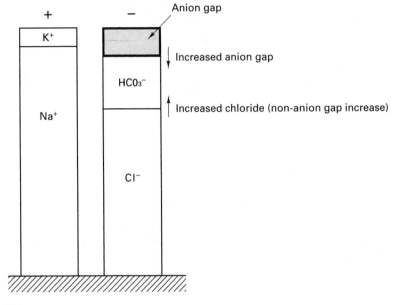

Fig. 2.52

- Lactic acidosis
- Ketoacidosis
- Renal failure (only when severe = creatinine > 0.4 mmol/l)
- Toxin ingestion – including salicylate, ethylene glycol, methanol

OSMOLAR GAP

Osmolality may be measured directly or can be calculated.

Calculated osmolality is derived by doubling the sodium and adding the glucose and urea:

$$2 \times (Na) + glucose + urea$$

Substances which may be present in the plasma in sufficient quantity to exert a significant osmotic effect but are not represented in the calculation, such as alcohol, mannitol and ethylene glycol, will result in an osmolar gap.

ELECTROLYTE DISTURBANCE – EXAMPLES

Hyperosmolality

An elderly lady is admitted unconscious to intensive care with the following electrolytes:

Sodium	156	(132–144 mmol/l)
Potassium	4.7	(3.1–4.8 mmol/l)
Chloride	128	(93–108 mmol/l)
Bicarbonate	25	(21–32 mmol/l)
Glucose	55	(3.0–5.5 mmol/l)
Urea	18.0	(3.0–8.0 mmol/l)
Creatinine	0.14	(0.06–0.12 mmol/l)
Measured osmolality	388	(280–295 mosmol/kg)

Osmolality may be measured directly or can be calculated.

Calculated osmolality is derived by doubling the sodium and adding the glucose and urea:

$$2 \times (Na) + glucose + urea$$

$$2 \times (156) + 55 + 18 = 385$$

Thus calculated and measured osmolality are similar: there is no gap.

Sometimes the measured osmolality will be higher than the calculated osmolality due to the presence of substances with osmotic activity (mannitol, ethylene glycol, alcohol).

This patient is in hyperosmolar diabetic coma.

Hypernatraemia

Following a severe head injury a 20-year-old man has the following electrolyte results:

Plasma

Sodium	165	(132–144 mmol/l)
Potassium	3.5	(3.1–4.8 mmol/l)
Chloride	126	(93–108 mmol/l)
Bicarbonate	23	(21–32 mmol/l)
Glucose	12.0	(3.0–5.5 mmol/l)
Measured osmolality	354	(280–295 mosmol/kg)

Urine

Sodium	< 5 mmol/l
Measured osmolality	124 mosmol/kg

This man has diabetes insipidus.

With such a high serum osmolality (i.e. too little serum water) he should be producing a hyperosmolar (concentrated urine) but he is not.

Diabetes mellitus causes urine to be highly osmolar because of the presence of glucose.

In ICU diabetes insipidus (DI) is usually seen in the setting of brain death. It is treated by replacement using DDAVP.

It is important to diagnose DI early before patients become dehydrated. Urine outputs of > 200 ml/h should cause suspicion of DI in brain-dead patients.

Hyperosmolality

A man is admitted unconscious to ICU following a head injury.
His electrolytes are as follows:

Plasma

Sodium	135	(132–144 mmol/l)
Potassium	4.0	(3.1–4.8 mmol/l)
Chloride	105	(93–108 mmol/l)
Bicarbonate	29	(21–32 mmol/l)
Glucose	5.0	(3.0–5.5 mmol/l)
Urea	4.0	(3.0–8.0 mmol/l)
Creatinine	0.06	(0.06–0.12 mmol/l)
Measured osmolality	350	(280–295 mosmol/kg)

Calculated osmolality = 279

Thus calculated is less than measured osmolality: there is a gap of 71.

This is due to the presence of substances with osmotic activity (mannitol, ethylene glycol, alcohol, methanol), in this case alcohol and mannitol.

Hyponatraemia

A 60-year-old lady suffers a convulsion 4 days after having a laparotomy for an aortic aneurysm repair. She suffered hypotension during her operation and has received 2000 ml 5% dextrose daily since her operation.
Her electrolytes are as follows:

Plasma

Sodium	109	(132–144 mmol/l)
Potassium	2.5	(3.1–4.8 mmol/l)
Chloride	77	(93–108 mmol/l)
Bicarbonate	25	(21–32 mmol/l)
Glucose	5.1	(3.0–5.5 mmol/l)
Urea	2.9	(3.0–8.0 mmol/l)
Creatinine	0.06	(0.06–0.12 mmol/l)
Measured osmolality	226	(280–295 mosmol/kg)

Urine

Sodium	43 mmol/l
Osmolality	253 mosmol/kg

This is iatrogenic water intoxication.

Diabetes insipidus and osmotic diuresis result in loss of free water from the body and hyperosmolality.

In this case there is excessive body free water. This excessive water is not being excreted by the kidney which is inappropriate.

Following surgical stress ADH secretion is increased (pain, morphine, etc. increase secretion) and water loads are excreted poorly – especially by women – so water loads as represented by 5% dextrose should be avoided or used with care.

Patients with hyponatraemia (particularly chronic) have subsequently developed severe neurological degeneration. While the relationship between treatment and neurological deterioration is unclear it is recommended that sodium levels are not increased at greater than 2 mmol/l/h or 25 mmol/l/d and that sodium levels are not permitted to overshoot (i.e. to become > 135 mmol/l).

Hyponatraemia

A man is admitted to the emergency department in a confused state. Examination reveals a normal state of hydration. He is on no diuretics.

His electrolytes are as follows:

Plasma

Sodium	116	(132–144 mmol/l)
Potassium	3.7	(3.1–4.8 mmol/l)
Chloride	81	(93–108 mmol/l)
Bicarbonate	25	(21–32 mmol/l)
Glucose	3.1	(3.0–5.5 mmol/l)
Urea	3.0	(3.0–8.0 mmol/l)
Creatinine	0.09	(0.06–0.12 mmol/l)
Measured osmolality	233	(280–295 mosmol/kg)

Urine

Sodium	83 mmol/l
Potassium	34 mmol/l
Osmolality	693 mosmol/kg

This is the syndrome of inappropriate ADH (SIADH).

This man has hyponatraemia with low osmolality. In this situation he would be expected to produce a urine of low osmolality to get rid of the water.

This is not the case. He is producing a urine with an osmolality greater than his serum osmolality which, in the face of hypo-osmolality, is inappropriate.

Beware making a diagnosis of SIADH in patients who are undervolumed or on diuretics.

SIADH is commonly caused by a bronchial carcinoma. Treatment is by treating the carcinoma and by water restriction.

ADH secretion is enhanced following surgery and by opiates. Water loading (e.g. 5% IV dextrose) should be avoided in this situation.

Hyponatraemia – hyperosmolar

An insulin-dependent diabetic with renal failure on chronic dialysis is admitted to ICU in a semi-conscious state.

Electrolyte results are as follows:

Sodium	93	(132–144 mmol/l)
Potassium	6.7	(3.1–4.8 mmol/l)
Chloride	58	(93–108 mmol/l)
Bicarbonate	16	(21–32 mmol/l)
Glucose	127	(3.0–5.5 mmol/l)
Urea	29.2	(3.0–8.0 mmol/l)
Creatinine	0.29	(0.06–0.12 mmol/l)
Measured osmolality	347	(280–295 mosmol/l)

This is hyperosmolar hyponatraemia. The low plasma sodium is due to intracellular to extracellular fluid shifts as a result of the high osmotic gradient (owing to her very high glucose) pulling water out of cells.

In hyperosmolar hyponatraemia an approximation of the 'true' sodium can be calculated by dividing the glucose by 4 and adding this to the measured sodium.

Non-anion gap metabolic acidosis

A patient with a high output small bowel fistula is referred to ICU due to increasing tachypnoea. His electrolytes and blood gas results show:

Sodium	130	(132–144 mmol/l)
Potassium	3.0	(3.1–4.8 mmol/l)
Chloride	108	(93–108 mmol/l)
Bicarbonate	15	(21–32 mmol/l)
Urea	20.2	(3.0–8.0 mmol/l)
Creatinine	0.14	(0.06–0.12 mmol/l)
pH	7.26	(7.35–7.42)
P_{CO_2}	4.27	(4.4–5.8 kPa)

This is hyperchloraemic non-anion gap acidosis.

There is an acidosis (pH = 7.26) but no increased anion gap (anion gap = 10).

Hyperchloraemic non-anion gap acidosis is caused by bicarbonate loss and/or chloride administration. Bicarbonate loss may be from the gut or kidneys.

In this case the likely cause is bicarbonate-rich fluid loss from the patient's small bowel fistula.

He needs fluid replacement with added potassium. Some bicarbonate is also appropriate since this has been lost.

Anion gap 1

The following results are received at 7 a.m. following an urgent request in a patient with an SVT of 160/min and a blood pressure of 90/65:

Sodium	133	(132–144 mmol/l)
Potassium	2.0	(3.1–4.8 mmol/l)

Chloride   110   (93–108 mmol/l)
Bicarbonate   31   (21–32 mmol/l)

These results must be incorrect. The anion gap is −6.

Negative anion gaps are not possible, so the results must be wrong.

Either a laboratory error (likely at 7 a.m. at changeover) or a transcription error has occurred.

Laboratory overestimation of chloride is the commonest cause.

Anion gap 2

A man is referred to intensive care because he is increasingly confused and his urine output has reduced.

His electrolytes are as follows:

Plasma

Sodium	138	(132–144 mmol/l)
Potassium	2.7	(3.1–4.8 mmol/l)
Chloride	71	(93–108 mmol/l)
Bicarbonate	45	(21–32 mmol/l)
Glucose	5.1	(3.0–5.5 mmol/l)
Urea	22.6	(3.0–8.0 mmol/l)
Creatinine	0.12	(0.06–0.12 mmol/l)

The high bicarbonate indicates a metabolic alkalosis. Metabolic alkalosis is common in sick patients because of potassium depletion (hydrogen ions enter cells to maintain electrical neutrality when K^+ is not available and bicarbonate remains extracellularly) and volume depletion (bicarbonate will be reabsorbed from the tubular fluid when sodium is maximally reabsorbed since there is inadequate chloride to be reabsorbed with all of the sodium).

There is an increased anion gap (25) which indicates a metabolic acidosis.

Note that both alkalosis and acidosis can coexist and in this case the pH may be normal even though the acid base status is grossly upset.

Volume depletion and a protein load in the bowel (usually blood) are the two main causes of a discrepancy between the urea and creatinine where the urea is higher than would be expected from the creatinine. In this case the creatinine is at the upper range of normality while the urea is more than twice normal.

This man had a colectomy and then developed an abdominal collection. The alkalosis is due to potassium and volume depletion and he then became very septic with a lactic acidosis.

Anion gap 3

A 20-year-old woman is brought to the emergency department having been found unconscious in her flat.

Her electrolyte and blood gas results are as follows:

Sodium	133	(132–144 mmol/l)
Potassium	2.6	(3.1–4.8 mmol/l)
Chloride	100	(93–108 mmol/l)
Bicarbonate	14	(21–32 mmol/l)
Glucose	8.3	(3.0–5.5 mmol/l)
Urea	12.7	(3.0–8.0 mmol/l)
Creatinine	0.19	(0.06–0.12 mmol/l)
Measured osmolality	290	(280–295 mosmol/kg)
pH	7.48	(7.35–7.42)
P_{CO_2}	2.53	(4.4–5.8 kPa)
P_{O_2}	12.8	(10–13.3 kPa)

This young woman has a large anion gap so has a metabolic acidosis due to one of the following:

- Lactic acidosis
- Ketoacidosis
- Renal failure (only when severe = creatinine > 0.4 mmol/l)
- Toxin ingestion – including salicylate, ethylene glycol, methanol

Salicylate has a direct stimulatory effect on the respiratory centre so the hyperventilation is greater than would be predicted as a compensation for the metabolic acidosis and results in a net alkalosis – as seen in this case.

In addition, if the acidosis was due to ingestion of methanol or ethylene glycol then there would be an osmolar gap which is not present here.

Anion gap 4

A 16-year-old boy is brought to the emergency department because he has become drowsy.

His electrolyte and blood gas results are as follows:

Sodium	123	(132–144 mmol/l)
Potassium	7.6	(3.1–4.8 mmol/l)
Chloride	80	(93–108 mmol/l)
Bicarbonate	4	(21–32 mmol/l)
Glucose	25.3	(3.0–5.5 mmol/l)
Urea	14.7	(3.0–8.0 mmol/l)
Creatinine	0.49	(0.06–0.12 mmol/l)
Urinary ketones	Positive	

This boy has a large anion gap so has a metabolic acidosis due to one of the following:

- Lactic acidosis
- Ketoacidosis

- Renal failure (only when severe = creatinine > 0.4 mmol/litre)
- Toxin ingestion – including salicylate, ethylene glycol, methanol

Ketones are positive and he is hyperglycaemic so a diagnosis of diabetic ketoacidosis is suggested by these results.

Note that the creatinine is higher than predicted by the urea. This suggests that the laboratory method for creatinine analysis is interfered with by ketones causing an artificially high result for creatinine. Urea may be a better indicator of hydration in diabetic ketoacidosis.

Anion Gap 5

A man with severe congestive cardiac failure and COAD (FEV_1 = 500 ml) is admitted to ICU with an acute exacerbation of his respiratory disease.

The following electrolyte and blood gas results are obtained:

Sodium	136	(132–144 mmol/l)
Potassium	4.0	(3.1–4.8 mmol/l)
Chloride	85	(93–108 mmol/l)
Bicarbonate	24	(21–32 mmol/l)
Glucose	6.3	(3.0–5.5 mmol/l)
Urea	12.7	(3.0–8.0 mmol/l)
Creatinine	0.22	(0.06–0.12 mmol/l)
pH	7.20	(7.35–7.42)
P_{CO_2}	8.27	(4.4–5.8 kPa)
P_{O_2}	8.53	(10–13.3 kPa)

This man has a metabolic acidosis, metabolic alkalosis and respiratory acidosis.

He is acidotic, as can be seen by looking at his pH, and this is both metabolic (increased anion gap = 31) and respiratory as his P_{CO_2} is above the normal range.

The bicarbonate is not as low as would be expected from the degree of the anion gap. The gap is increased by 19 (31 minus the normal gap of about 12) and the bicarbonate level is usually reduced by the same amount as the gap is increased.

If his bicarbonate started at 30 then we would expect a level of 11 (30 – 19) with this degree of acidosis. In this case the bicarbonate before the acidosis developed must have been 24 + 19 = 43, a marked metabolic alkalosis, probably a result of his diuretic therapy but possibly also a consequence of compensation for CO_2 retention.

This is an example of 'triple' acid base disturbance.

Rhabdomyolysis

A woman is admitted to hospital having been found unconscious at her home. She is suspected to have taken a drug overdose.

Her electrolytes are as follows:

Plasma

Sodium	142	(132–144 mmol/l)
Potassium	6.9	(3.1–4.8 mmol/l)
Chloride	106	(93–108 mmol/l)
Bicarbonate	24	(21–32 mmol/l)
Glucose	5.8	(3.0–5.5 mmol/l)
Urea	15.0	(3.0–8.0 mmol/l)
Creatinine	0.16	(0.06–0.12 mmol/l)
Calcium	1.84	(2.05–2.55 mmol/l)
Phosphate	1.99	(0.60–1.25 mmol/l)
Albumin	40	(30–50 gm/l)
Urate	0.92	(0.12–0.45 mmol/l)

This is rhabdomyolysis.

The high phosphate, potassium and urate are all markers of cell lysis. The low calcium is due to binding of plasma calcium to myofibrils consequent upon muscle cell lysis.

Rhabdomyolysis is described as a complication of many drugs in overdose or may occur as a consequence of prolonged immobility on the ground and pressure effect. In this case the CK was > 100000 U.

HAEMODYNAMIC CALCULATIONS

SV: stroke volume

SV (in ml) = (CO/HR) × 1000.

SI (in ml/m^2) = SB/BSA.

Definition
The stroke volume is calculated by dividing the cardiac output by the heart rate. Multiplying this value by the conversion factor of 1000 changes litres into millilitres. Stroke volume measures the amount of blood ejected by the ventricle with each cardiac contraction.

Significance
Normal stoke volume is 60–70 ml (normal range for stroke index is 41–51 ml/m^2). The stroke volume depends on factors affecting the ventricular muscle, preload, afterload and contractility.

Stroke volume may be affected by factors influencing total blood volume and central venous return, resistance to forward systolic ejection of the blood in the ventricle, and the contractile state of the myocardium. Increased stroke volume is associated with bradycardia and positive inotropic agents which increase contractility. Stroke volume also increases rapidly at the beginning of exercise and usually plateaus at near maximal values before less than half of maximal exercise capacity is reached.

SVR: systemic vascular resistance

SVR (in dynes $\times$ s/cm^5) = 79.96 $\times$ (ABPm – CVP)/CO.

SVRI (in dynes $\times$ s/cm^5) $\times$ m^2) = SVR $\times$ BSA.

Definition

Systemic vascular resistance measures the load applied to the left ventricular muscle during ventricular ejection. Vascular resistance to blood flow is calculated by analogy to Ohm's law: the resistance in a circuit is equal to the voltage across the circuit divided by the current

$$\text{Resistance} = \frac{\text{voltage difference}}{\text{current flow}}$$

$$\text{Resistance} = \frac{\text{mean pressure differential across vascular bed}}{\text{blood flow}}$$

The pressure difference between the proximal and distal ends of the cardiovascular system (arterial and venous) is divided by the cardiac output. This value is multiplied by the conversion factor which changes resistance units of mmHg/l/min to dynes $\times$ s/cm^5.

Significance

Normal SVR is 770–1500 dynes $\times$ s/cm^5 (normally SVRI is 1970–2390 (dynes $\times$ s/cm^5) $\times$ m^2).

Vascular resistance increases when arterioles constrict, increasing the load against which the ventricle must pump. Increased SVR is associated with vasoconstriction, left ventricular failure, hypovolaemic shock, cardiogenic shock, inotropic agents and increased blood viscosity, as with polycythaemia vera.

Decreased SVR may be due to vasodilation (commonly sepsis), moderate hypoxaemia, vasodilators or decreased blood viscosity as with anaemia.

PVR: pulmonary vascular resistance

PVR (in dynes $\times$ s/cm^5) = 79.96 $\times$ (PAPm – PAWP)/CO.

PVRI (in dynes $\times$ s/cm^5) $\times$ m^2) = PVR $\times$ BSA.

Definition

Pulmonary vascular resistance is an index of the resistance offered by the pulmonary capillaries to the systolic effort of the right ventricle. As with SVR, PVR is calculated by analogy to Ohm's law, by deriving the pressure differential between the mean pulmonary arterial pressure and the pulmonary artery wedge pressure and dividing that value by the cardiac output.

Significance

Normal PVR is 100–250 dynes $\times$ s/cm^5. Normal PVRI is 225–315 (dynes $\times$ s/cm^5) $\times$ m^2.

Under normal circumstances, the pulmonary vascular resistance is one-sixth that of the systemic vascular bed. Pulmonary vascular disease is associated with increased PVR which may exceed SVR.

Increased PVR is related to alveolar hypoxia which causes vasoconstriction of the precapillary pulmonary arterioles.

In normal lungs, pulmonary artery pressures do not increase until approximately two-thirds of the lung vessels are obstructed. Mitral stenosis, pulmonary oedema and obliteration of the pulmonary capillary bed also result in increased PVR.

LCW: left cardiac work

LCW (in kg $\times$ m) = CO $\times$ ABPm $\times$ 0.0136.

LCWI (in kg $\times$ m/m^2) = LCW/BSA.

Definition

Work is measured as the product of a force and the distance moved by the point of application of that force. In terms of cardiac work:

Work = pressure generated $\times$ volume of blood pumped

LCW measures the amount of work the left ventricle does each minute when ejecting blood. Atrial work is not included because of the relatively small pressures involved. Left cardiac work is calculated as the product of the mean arterial blood pressure and the cardiac output.

The conversion factor of 0.0136 converts mmHg to kg $\times$ m.

Significance

Normal LCWI is 3.4–4.2 kg $\times$ m/m^2. Left cardiac work increases or decreases with changes in either pressure (arterial blood pressure) or volume (cardiac output).

LVSW: left ventricular stroke work

LVSW (in g $\times$ m) = SV $\times$ ABPm $\times$ 0.0136.

LVSWI (in g $\times$ m/m^2) = LVSM/BSA.

Definition

LVSW is a measure of the amount of work the left ventricle does per beat:

Work = pressure generated $\times$ volume of blood pumped.

LVSW is calculated as the product of the mean arterial pressure and the stroke volume. The conversion factor of 0.0136 again converts ml $\times$ mmHg to g $\times$ m.

Significance
Normal LVSWI is 50–62 g × m/m². LVSWI is an assessment of contractility. A low or decreasing LVSWI may indicate a requirement for an inotropic agent to strengthen cardiac contraction.

RCW: right cardiac work

RCW (in kg × m) = CO × PAPm × 0.0136.

RCWI (in kg × m/m²) = RCW/BSA.

Definition
In a similar way to the LCW, RCW measures the work that the right ventricle does each minute when ejecting blood. It is calculated as the product of the mean pulmonary artery pressure and the cardiac output.

Significance
Normal RCWI is 0.54–0.66 kg × m/m². As with left cardiac work, RCW increases or decreases with changes in pressure (pulmonary artery pressure) or volume (cardiac output).

RVSW: right ventricular stroke work

RVSW (in g × m) = SV × PAPm × 0.0136.

RVSWI (in g × m/m²) = RVSW/BSA.

Definition
RVSW measures the amount of work the right ventricle does per beat when ejecting blood, similarly to the left ventricular stroke work measurement. It is calculated as the product of the mean pulmonary artery pressure and the stroke volume.

Significance
Normal RVSWI is 7.9–9.7 g × m/m². As with left ventricular stroke work, RVSW is a measure of the heart's pumping performance (myocardial contractility).

Haemodynamic profiles (examples)

CI	2.15 l/min/m²	2.5–4.0	*Low*
SVRI	2707 dyn.s.m²/cm⁵	1970–2390	*High*
PVRI	271 dyn.s.m²/cm⁵	225–315	
LVSWI	25.0 g.m/m²	50–62	*Low*
CVP	8 mmHg		
PAWP	18 mmHg		*High*

A picture of low cardiac output, high systemic vascular resistance and low left ventricular stroke work index (LVSWI) is characteristic of cardiogenic shock due to left ventricular failure.

CI	$1.85 l/min/m^2$	Low
SVRI	$3227 dyn.s.m^2/cm^5$	High
PVRI	$271 dyn.s.m^2/cm^5$	
LVSWI	$17.0 g.m/m^2$	Low
CVP	$24 mmHg$	High
PAWP	$6 mmHg$	Low

A picture of low cardiac output, high systemic vascular resistance and low left ventricular stroke work index (LVSWI) with a high CVP but a low PAWP is characteristic of cardiogenic shock due to right ventricular failure.

Right ventricular infarction should be suspected in those with shock following inferior infarction. Fluid loading is often remarkably effective.

CI	$3.15 l/min/m^2$	High
SVRI	$707 dyn.s.m^2/cm^5$	Low
PVRI	$371 dyn.s.m^2/cm^5$	
LVSWI	$31.0 g.m/m^2$	Low
CVP	$6 mmHg$	Low
PAWP	$9 mmHg$	Low

A picture of high cardiac output, low systemic vascular resistance and somewhat low left ventricular stroke work index (LVSWI) is characteristic of septic shock.

Although contractility is reduced (sometimes markedly) cardiac output is usually increased or maintained because afterload is reduced.

OXYGEN CALCULATIONS

In the critically ill patient, an adequate oxygenation system is essential for recovery. The oxygenation calculations help characterize the efficiency of the oxygenation of blood and the rates of oxygen delivery and consumption.

S_vO_2: mixed venous oxygen saturation

Definition

The saturation of blood returning from the tissues which has been mixed as a consequence of right heart contraction (blood from the superior vena cava, inferior vena cava and cardiac sinus have differing saturations) and is sampled from the pulmonary artery.

Significance

Under normal circumstances only a proportion of the oxygen carried by the blood is released during passage through the tissues and the mixed venous saturation is about 75%. In low flow states increased tissue extraction results in a low S_vO_2. Identification of a low S_vO_2 either by continuous monitoring, using a pulmonary artery catheter with a fibreoptic tip, or by intermittent blood sampling indicates inadequate tissue perfusion.

C_aO_2: arterial oxygen content

C_aO_2 (in ml/100 ml) = $(1.34 \times [Hb] \times S_aO_2/100) + (P_aO_2 \times 0.0031)$.

Definition

The oxygen content of blood is divided between the oxygen bound to haemoglobin and the small amount of oxygen dissolved in blood. The concentration of bound oxygen is calculated using the number of grams of haemoglobin per 100 ml of blood (HGB) and the percentage oxyhaemoglobin saturation (S_aO_2). One gram of saturated haemoglobin binds 1.34 millilitres of oxygen. Each millimetre of mercury (mmHg) of oxygen partial pressure corresponds to an oxygen concentration of 0.0031 ml/100 ml. The total oxygen content is the sum of the bound and unbound oxygen concentrations.

Significance

Normal range for C_aO_2 readings is 17–20 ml/100 ml of blood. Abnormally low values suggest a low haemoglobin content or inefficient gas exchange in the lungs.

C_vO_2: venous oxygen content

C_vO_2 (in ml/100 ml) = $(1.34 \times [Hb] \times S_vO_2/100) + (P_vO_2 \times 0.0031)$.

Definition

The C_vO_2 is a measure of the oxygen content of venous blood. The formula is similar to the formula for C_aO_2 and has essentially the same explanation.

Significance

Normal values for C_vO_2 range from 12 to 15 ml/dl. Tissues receiving a markedly reduced blood flow will extract oxygen more completely which may be reflected in abnormally low values of C_vO_2, and abnormally high values for $_{av}DO_2$ and O_2ER.

$_{av}DO_2$: arteriovenous oxygen difference

$_{av}D_aO_2$ (in ml/dl) = $C_aO_2 - C_vO_2$.

Definition

The $_{av}DO_2$ is the amount of oxygen that, at the time of arterial and venous blood sampling, left the systemic capillaries to be consumed in the tissues.

Significance
Arterial blood normally has 4.2–5.0 ml more oxygen per 100 ml of blood than does venous blood. Abnormally high values may reflect more complete extraction of oxygen from the blood, as is characteristic in tissues receiving decreased blood flow. This occurs during shock, when blood is preferentially diverted to the brain and heart. Values greater than approximately 5.6 ml/100 ml are reason for serious concern. In such a situation the oxygen extraction ratio (O_2ER) will also be abnormally high.

O_2AV: oxygen availability

O_2AV (ml/min) = $C_aO_2 \times Co \times 10$.

O_2AVI ((ml/min)/m^2) = O_2AV/BSA.

Definition
The oxygen content of the blood is multiplied by the cardiac output to give a measure of the rate of oxygen delivery to the tissues. The factor of 10 converts to decility. O_2AV expresses the amount of oxygen delivered to the systemic capillaries and therefore potentially 'available' to the tissues.

Significance
This variable helps determine whether a patient's heart and lungs are operating efficiently enough to make an adequate amount of oxygen available to the tissues. The normal range of O_2AV is 950–1150 ml/min (O_2AVI 550–650 (ml/min)/m^2).

Therapeutic manipulations which increase O_2AVI are considered beneficial in septic shock.

Vo_2: oxygen consumption

Vo_2 (ml/min) = $_{av}Do_2 \times Co \times 10$.

Vo_2I ((ml/min)/m^2) = Vo_2/BSA.

Definition
$_{av}Do_2$ is multiplied by the cardiac output to yield Vo_2, a measure of the rate of oxygen consumption by the tissues over time.

Significance
Normal Vo_2 range 195–285 ml/min. Vo_2I is 115–165 ml/min/m^2. In critically ill patients higher values, 150–200 ml/min/m^2, are desirable. Low values of Vo_2I indicate that the metabolic needs of the tissues are not being met.

In septic shock increasing oxygen availability is generally associated with an increased oxygen consumption.

N.B. Beware using derived saturations from blood gas machines for calculating oxygen delivery and consumption. Values have been shown to be inaccurate and when this variation is combined with errors inherent in cardiac output measurement the calculated values for oxygen delivery and consumption have been shown to be very unreliable. Directly measured saturations using a co-oximeter are required for reliable values to be produced.

O_2ER: oxygen extraction ratio

$O_2ER = (C_aO_2 - C_vO_2)/C_aO_2$.

Definition
This is the ratio of oxygen consumption to oxygen availability (VO_2/O_2AV). This ratio simplifies to the above formula when the formulas for VO_2 and O_2AV are substituted in and common factors divided out.

Significance
The O_2ER is the fraction of available oxygen that is extracted and consumed by the tissues. The normal range is 0.24–0.28. Values greater than 0.35 indicate significantly inadequate oxygen delivery to tissues.

$_{Aa}DO_2$: alveolar–arterial oxygen difference

$_{Aa}DO_2$ (in mmHg) = P_AO_2

where $P_AO_2 = F_iO_2 \times (PB - 47) - P_aCO_2$.

Definition
The $_{Aa}DO_2$ measures the difference in partial pressure of oxygen between the alveoli and the arteries. $_{Aa}DO_2$ reflects the efficiency of oxygen exchange between the lung alveoli and the pulmonary capillaries.

P_AO_2 is calculated using the barometric pressure (PB), the partial pressure of saturated water pressure at 37°C (47 mmHg). The fraction of inspired oxygen (F_iO_2), and the partial pressure of carbon dioxide in arterial blood (P_aCO_2).

P_ACO_2 is assumed to be approximately equal to P_aCO_2.

Significance
Normal $_{Aa}DO_2$ is 10–15 mmHg for patients breathing room air and 10–65 mmHg for patients breathing 100% oxygen.

Qs/Qt: percentage arteriovenous shunt

$$Qs/Qt = \frac{100 \times 1.34 \times [Hb] + 0.0031 \times P_AO_2 - C_aO_2}{1.34 \times [Hb] + 0.003 \times P_AO_2 - C_vO_2}$$

Definition
Some venous blood bypasses the pulmonary capillaries. In healthy individuals venous return from the bronchial arteries and some from the coro-

nary circulation flows to the left heart without being oxygenated. In sick patients, an additional volume of blood in the pulmonary circulation remains deoxygenated by flowing either through poorly ventilated alveoli or through areas of alveolar-capillary block.

Significance
Qs/Qt is a measure of the efficiency of pulmonary oxygenation. Normal Qs/Qt is low. Values of 15 suggest moderate lung dysfunction and values of 30 indicate severe pulmonary dysfunction.

Viva questions

The viva forms a crucial part of the FRCA examination. Each viva consists of being asked questions by two examiners across a table. Responses should be well structured and confidently presented. The guidance given at the start of the 'Answer Plan' section and the plans themselves will help give you an indication of how to structure your responses. Presentation improves with practice and candidates should enlist the help of senior colleagues to give them practice vivas. This may not always be possible, so a number of specimen questions are given on the following pages. To obtain maximum benefit these are best answered orally in a 'mock viva' situation with a colleague asking the questions. The importance of using every chance to practise viva technique cannot be overemphasized since it is surprisingly difficult to give good oral answers, even on topics with which you are familiar. An example viva answer is included (p. 229).

Viva 1

1. Describe the anaesthetic management of a 50-year-old man with diffuse submandibular cellulitis and an abscess requiring incision and drainage
2. Draw the laryngeal opening. What is the nerve supply?
3. Describe the anaesthetic management of a 7-year-old child with a full stomach and a penetrating eye injury
4. Tell me about the pharmacology of atracurium. Who was Hoffmann?
5. What is the effect of smoke exposure in a house fire? How would you assess and manage an exposed patient?
6. What is the pathophysiology of ARDS? How is it treated? What is meant by 'best PEEP'?
7. Compare desflurane and sevoflurane. What are the advantages of desflurane over other agents? What are its disadvantages?

Viva 2

1. What is Sellick's manoeuvre? How else can you manage a patient with a full stomach?
2. Do you think we should stop using suxamethonium? What are its advantages? What are the problems with it? Is vecuronium then ideal?
3. What would you do if a child had a tense jaw and did not seem to relax well after being given suxamethonium? What are the features of malignant hyperpyrexia? Does previous uncomplicated halothane exposure exclude the diagnosis?
4. Does a history of epilepsy influence your anaesthetic management?
5. What percentage of the available volatile agents is metabolized? What are the metabolic products? Which agents produce fluoride? What is the danger of fluoride?
6. You are using thiopental with a new SHO who has never seen it before; what would you tell him about it? Can you draw the formula? How does methohexitone differ?
7. What do you understand by structure activity relationships? Can you explain the differences in activity with catecholamines? How about volatile agents?

Viva 3

1. What are the possible causes of a patient not breathing at the end of an operation? How can you differentiate between these causes? How do you demonstrate that a patient has atypical cholinesterase? How would you manage a patient homozygous for atypical cholinesterase who was apnoeic after suxamethonium?
2. What types of allergy do you know? What sorts most commonly complicate anaesthesia?
3. How do you establish brain death? Who laid down these guidelines? What must you exclude before these tests can be validly performed?
4. Do you use blood filters? What types are there? When would you use one? Why do you not always use one when giving blood?
5. What are the problems of massive blood transfusion? What are ACD, CPD and SAGM blood? What the differences between them considering the factors that are deficient? What is the potassium concentration in 3-week-old stored blood?
6. How would you perform local anaesthesia for a bronchoscopy?
7. What did John Snow contribute to anaesthesia?

Viva 4

1. When do you think a PAFC might be helpful? How is it inserted? What are the pressures which you encounter as it is advanced? What are the risks?
2. How would you anaesthetize a child for a bronchoscopy?

3. When might you use an Ambu E valve? Draw me a 'draw-over' anaesthetic system. Why do we not use draw-over systems more often? What are the disadvantages of nitrous oxide?

4. What are the MAC, boiling point and saturated vapour pressure of halothane? What concentration of isoflurane would you achieve if you put it in a halothane vaporizer set at 1.5%?

5. What factors predispose patients to electrocution? What is microshock? How do you protect patients from these risks?

6. Can you draw me the Mapleson classification of breathing systems? What sort of circuit is a Bain circuit? What are its advantages and disadvantages? What fresh gas flow do you need to prevent CO_2 rebreathing?

7. What is Laplace's law? Can you think of any applications of this in anaesthesia?

Viva 5

1. Draw a circle system for me. What are the effects of having the vaporizer in circuit or outside circuit? How does soda lime work? What are the benefits of a circle system?

2. What features would you desire in an endotracheal tube for intensive care use?

3. Draw the sensory pathways in the spinal cord. How does a cordotomy help relieve pain?

4. What are the possible complications of epidurals in labour?

5. How would you perform a regional block for a hernia repair in a patient who cannot have a spinal or epidural? What about for a laparotomy?

6. Features of a Robert–Shaw tube. How do you conduct one-lung anaesthesia? How can the hypoxia be minimized?

7. Name the foramina in the skull. What passes through each?

Viva 6

1. How would you manage a case of suspected epiglottitis in a child of 6 years?

2. Do you use hypotension in anaesthesia? When would you use it and why? How do you manage such a case?

3. What is the natural history of an extradural haematoma? What are the principles of anaesthesia for a patient with an expanding intracranial haematoma?

4. What are the causes of postoperative hypoxia?

5. You are going to use this Boyle's machine; can you show me how you would check it?

6. When might you use helium? What formula explains why it helps in this situation?

7. What sort of flowmeter is a rotameter? What sources of inaccuracies are there with rotameters?

Viva 7

1. Are you ever asked to look at the cords after thyroidectomy? What might you see? What is the innervation of the larynx? What is the effect of complete section or partial damage to either of these nerves? What is Semon's law?
2. What do you know about opioid receptors? What is a partial agonist?
3. How many centimetres of water is pipeline pressure? Show me where pressure is reduced as the gas passes through the Boyle's machine? What safety features are present to prevent barotrauma?
4. You are asked to anaesthetize a man who suffered a C8/T1 cord lesion one month previously, for a cystoscopy. What are the problems associated with this and how would you manage such a case?
5. Do you have a 'failed intubation drill'? Describe it to me.
6. Show me how you would perform a brachial plexus block. What are the risks of this method? Do you know another approach?
7. Do you ever give caudals? What precautions do you take? How do you calculate the dose/volume?

Viva 8

1. You are called to see a 60-year-old man with a flail chest; how would you assess him? How would you manage such a case?
2. You are asked to anaesthetize a 3 kg baby with pyloric stenosis; how would you manage it?
3. What do you understand by IMV, MMV, HFJV, pH, PEEP, CPAP?
4. What are the problems inherent in obesity from the anaesthetic point of view? What is pickwickian syndrome?
5. How would you anaesthetize a patient with a bronchopleural fistula?
6. Have you ever used a draw-over anaesthetic system? What features would you desire in a vaporizer for use in a draw-over system? What are the advantages of a draw-over system? Have you heard of the 'Triservice' system?

Viva 9

1. Can you draw me a diagram to show me what the pin index system for medical gases looks like? What is the 'washer' called? Do you know the pin positions for oxygen, nitrous oxide and cyclopropane?
2. What colour cylinders are the different medical gases in? What pressures are they under? How much oxygen is there in a size E cylinder? What is the Poynting effect? If you had an Entonox cylinder in your car boot overnight in a cold winter, how would you ensure that your patient received a correct mixture?

3. What are the problems associated with anaesthesia for carotid endarterectomy?
4. If money was no object, which ventilator would you like for use in theatre? What are the attractive features of this ventilator?
5. How do you diagnose tracheo-oesophageal fistula? What are the anaesthetic considerations of this condition?
6. What do you know about opioid receptors? What is enkephalin? What is endorphin? At which receptors does morphine act?
7. How would you perform an ankle block for an avulsion of an ingrowing great toe nail? What other nerves are there at the ankle?

Viva 10

1. What evidence is there that trace concentrations of anaesthetic agents are harmful? What ways of scavenging do you know?
2. Draw a vitalograph trace which you might expect from a patient with obstructive lung disease. Now draw one from a patient with a restrictive defect. What other useful tests of preoperative respiratory function do you know?
3. What sort of preoperative lung function test results predict postoperative respiratory failure? How would you manage a patient with such results for a hysterectomy?
4. Describe the anaesthetic management of a patient for a renal transplant.
5. What causes do you consider when recovery from anaesthesia is delayed? What tests can you perform to help you decide?
6. Have you read any paper over the last year which has significantly influenced your anaesthetic practice?
7. How do NSAIDs work? What side-effects do they have? Explain the difference between COX1 and COX2 inhibitors?

Viva 11

1. How can you assess reversal from neuromuscular blockade? What is TOF and TOF ratio? Explain post tetanic facilitation. What is a tetanic stimulus and what is its use?
2. What clinical signs would suggest air embolism during anaesthesia? How can it happen? Where are the danger areas in neurosurgery? How would you detect it and how would you treat it?
3. What is massive blood transfusion? What complications can occur with massive transfusion? How would you manage a patient with major haemorrhage?
4. What is malignant hyperpyrexia? What are the early signs? How would you treat it? How would you manage the MH sensitive patient?
5. How would you anaesthetize a patient for microlaryngoscopy? What is a Carden tube and how is it used? What are the dangers of this technique?

6. What is pulsus parodoxus? Where would you meet this? How would you anaesthetize a patient with cardiac tamponade?
7. How would you manage a patient with status epilepticus? What would happen if such a patient were given muscle relaxants? How would you monitor this patient if paralysed and ventilated?

Viva 12

1. Describe your initial management of a patient admitted with burns? How much fluid would you give this patient? What fluid would you give this patient? How would you monitor fluid replacement?
2. A patient collapses as you inject an induction dose of sodium thiopental – how would you manage this case? What is the incidence of anaphylaxis from thiopental? How severe is it? Which drugs can be administered via the endotracheal tube?
3. How would you manage a case of severe asthma who requires IPPV? What drugs would you use to facilitate intubation? What would you use to sedate the patient? Would you paralyse the patient?
4. Which techniques of central venous cannulation do you use? What are the complications associated with inserting a subclavian line and an internal jugular line? How would you insert a central line in a patient with a clotting problem?
5. What is a pulmonary artery flotation catheter? What are the indications for its use? What can you directly measure with one? What measurements can be derived? What equipment is necessary for this?
6. A patient develops fast atrial fibrillation whilst under anaesthesia – what would you do if the patient was severely hypotensive? Which drugs could you use? If the patient was an elderly lady undergoing hip surgery under a spinal anaesthetic, what would you do?
7. Does calcium have any part to play in resuscitation during a cardiac arrest? What is the role of adrenaline (epinephrine) and sodium bicarbonate? What would you do for a patient with complete heart block? What techniques of pacing do you know about? Which drug could you use in this situation? How would you administer it? How can you recognize complete heart block in a patient with a ventricular rate of 60?

Viva 13

1. How would you replace potassium in a severely hypokalaemic patient prior to urgent surgery? What are the dangers? How would you monitor the patient?
2. What is the normal level of potassium? What are the causes of hyperkalaemia? How can hyperkalaemia be treated? What is the effect of giving sodium bicarbonate?

3. A patient is admitted with a core temperature of 27°C – how would you manage this patient? What methods of rewarming could you use? Are there any dangers associated with rewarming? Should it be performed slowly or quickly? What associated factors should one consider in a patient admitted with hypothermia?
4. How would you manage a patient with an overdose of tricyclic antidepressants? What is the significance of ingestion of paracetamol with tricyclics?
5. How would you manage a patient with a paracetamol overdose? How does paracetamol damage the liver? How can this be prevented? What is the management of a patient who is seen too late for this treatment?
6. How would you manage a hypertensive patient in the postoperative period?
7. How would you manage a patient with pre-eclampsia who was being induced? How would you control the patient's blood pressure? How would you prevent seizures? How would you monitor the patient? How would you administer the drugs?

Viva 14

1. What are the problems associated with digoxin toxicity? What arrhythmias may be seen? What are the signs on the ECG? What are the ECG signs of hypokalaemia?
2. What are the problems associated with the lithotomy position? Are there any particular problems associated with spinal anaesthesia and this position? What happens at the end of the procedure? What problems can this cause?
3. Describe the autonomic nervous system? What are the transmitters? What is the effect of the parasympathetic nervous system on the heart, eyes and gut?
4. What is the Valsalva manoeuvre? Describe the changes that take place. Why might you ask a patient to perform this technique? What would you look for?
5. What sort of filters are used in anaesthesia? What size are they? When would you consider using a blood filter? What types are there?
6. Why are anaesthetic gases dry? What effect does dry gas have on the airways? How can we humidify anaesthetic gases in theatre?
7. What techniques for identifying the epidural space do you know? Describe a Tuohy needle. Do you use test doses? What are the advantages and disadvantages of test doses?

Viva 15

1. What is the composition of Hartmann's solution? Why do we use 5% dextrose? Name a plasma expander. What is it made of? How long does it stay in the circulation? What is the incidence of anaphylaxis with this expander?

2. What is the composition of soda lime? Why does there need to be water present? What are the reactions that take place? What are the advantages of circle anaesthesia? Why was circle anaesthesia popular in the early years of anaesthesia?
3. Which name is associated with 'to and fro' absorption anaesthesia? What are the disadvantages of this technique?
4. What is the hepatorenal syndrome? When may it develop? How can you prevent it?
5. How would you assess a patient's fitness to undergo day surgery? What are the contraindications? Are there any social contraindications?
6. How long after an anaesthetic would you recommend a patient did not drive? Why? How can you assess effects on cognitive function following anaesthesia?
7. What is the mechanism of the hypertensive response to intubation? In which particular cases is it most dangerous? How can it be obtunded?

Viva 16

1. How would you manage a patient for thyroidectomy? What are the particular dangers peroperatively and postoperatively? What is a thyroid storm? How would you manage it?
2. What is MAC? How is it affected by the age of the patient? What effect does nitrous oxide have on the MAC of a volatile agent?
3. What are the problems with using nitrous oxide? Is there any surgery where its use is contraindicated? Are there any patient problems that would contraindicate the use of nitrous oxide?
4. What is the second gas effect? Explain why we use overpressure. What is diffusion hypoxia?
5. How can you assess intubation difficulty preoperatively? How can you describe the degree of intubation difficulty at laryngoscopy?
6. Describe the nerve supply of the larynx? How would you perform an awake intubation? When might you use this technique?
7. Where is the site of action of opioids administered by the epidural route? Are there any dangers associated with this route of administration? What factors can increase the likelihood of problems?

Viva 17

1. How would you assess a patient prior to hypotensive anaesthesia? How would you monitor the patient? What techniques of hypotensive anaesthesia do you know?
2. What agent would you use for a gaseous induction? Why? When would you consider using a gaseous induction?
3. What are the features of aspirin overdose? How does it affect body pH? How is it treated? How does alkaline diuresis work?

4. How would you anaesthetize an 80-year-old lady with a fractured neck of femur? Is there any evidence of a difference in outcome between general anaesthesia and spinals?
5. How would you manage a patient you have intubated and ventilated who develops bronchospasm at the start of surgery?
6. What is a vapour? What is a gas? Which anaesthetic agents are vapours?
7. Describe how you would perform an axillary block. Does it provide uniform analgesia over the whole arm? Which nerves are most likely to be missed and why?

Viva 18

1. What are the factors that control intracranial pressure? How can you measure ICP? How can you control ICP? What are the dangers of using mannitol?
2. What factors influence the development of a spinal headache? How would you manage a dural puncture during insertion of an epidural? How would you manage a patient with a spinal headache?
3. What are the disadvantages of endotracheal intubation? How can you confirm correct placement of an endotracheal tube? Is capnography useful on other occasions?
4. During a neurosurgical operation your patient becomes desaturated and the capnograph shows low $ETco_2$ – what would you do? Where are the danger areas for this problem? What other monitor can be used to detect this problem? In a high-risk procedure what precautions would you take?
5. What would be the maximum pressure you could record at the common gas outlet? What is the function of the pressure-limiting valve? How are patients protected from barotrauma? What law explains the pressure changes in a reservoir bag?
6. What factors do you consider when positioning a patient on the operating table? Where are there particular dangers of nerve damage?
7. Explain the advantages and disadvantages of the Bain circuit. What gas flow do you need to use for spontaneous respiration and IPPV? Explain the technique of using this circuit for IPPV. What is an isopleth?

Viva 19

1. What ventilator do you use routinely in theatre? How does it work? What safety features does it have?
2. What are the signs of malignant hyperthermia? What is the inheritance and incidence of this condition? How would you manage such a case? How can you test for the condition?

3. What are the possible complications of intravenous regional anaesthesia? Describe how you would perform a Bier's block. What agent would you use? What are the problems associated with the use of bupivacaine? How can you treat dysrhythmias induced by bupivacaine?

4. What would you look for in the preoperative assessment of a 20-year-old with Down's syndrome? What about problems associated with intubation? For what procedures would you consider antibiotic prophylaxis in a patient with an abnormal heart valve? What would you give?

5. What are the problems associated with advanced rheumatoid arthritis? What tests would you like performed preoperatively on such a patient who requires an elective hip replacement? How would you manage this patient in the presence of an unstable neck?

6. Which non-invasive blood pressure monitor do you use? How does it work? What are its limitations?

7. Draw the oxygen dissociation curve. Why is it that shape? Which factors shift the curve to the right?

Viva 20

1. How would you define massive haemorrhage? How would you manage a case of massive haemorrhage in an obstetric patient? What are the hazards associated with massive blood transfusion?

2. A 20-year-old elective caesarean section patient at term becomes profoundly hypotensive soon after induction of general anaesthesia – what is your differential diagnosis? What would you do?

3. What are the major causes of maternal mortality? What are the main anaesthetic factors?

4. Describe the blood supply of the spinal cord. Describe the venous drainage.

5. You are presented with a patient for an elective hip replacement who is found to have a blood pressure of 180/115 and is on no medication – what would you do? What blood pressure would you accept prior to elective surgery? Why do you refuse to anaesthetize hypertensive patients? What would you do if it was an emergency operation?

6. Describe the blood supply of the left ventricle. When does it mostly occur? Which factors affect myocardial blood supply and demand? Which are the most important? What is the rate pressure product? How useful is it?

7. What ventilator do you use in the intensive care unit in your hospital? Describe how it works. What modes of ventilation does it allow? What would you look for in a paediatric ventilator?

Viva 21

1. You are referred an insulin-dependent diabetic for elective major surgery – what would you look for in your preoperative visit? What

tests would be useful? How would you manage the patient's diabetes on the day of surgery?

2. What is the difference between a right-sided and a left-sided Robert–Shaw tube? Which would you wish to use routinely for thoracic surgery and why? How do you ensure the correct positioning of this tube?

3. How would you anaesthetize a patient for rigid bronchoscopy? What is apnoeic oxygenation? How fast does the $P_a\text{CO}_2$ rise in an apnoeic patient?

4. What is the danger of using adrenaline (epinephrine) during anaesthesia? Which volatile agent is the safest when adrenaline (epinephrine) is being administered? What is the maximum dose you would allow to be administered?

5. How is carbon dioxide carried in the blood? Explain the effect of a raised carbon dioxide level on pH.

6. What assessment scales do you know about? Tell me about the Glasgow Coma Scale. What is the APACHE score? What is the use of this score?

7. What are the problems associated with anaesthetizing someone with aortic stenosis? What should be avoided in these patients?

Viva 22

1. What sort of laryngoscope would you use to intubate a neonate? Describe it. Why would you use this type of laryngoscope? How would you assess what size of endotracheal tube to use for an infant? Would you use a cuffed tube? Why did you give that answer? What other physiological differences are there compared to adults?

2. How would you describe to a colleague how to perform cricoid pressure? Who developed this technique? Why do we use the cricoid cartilage?

3. Describe the anatomy of the bronchial tree. Where do inhaled foreign bodies commonly lodge? What are the symptoms and signs seen in a child with an inhaled foreign body? What might you see on chest X-ray? How would you anaesthetize a child for bronchoscopic removal of a foreign body?

4. What type of circuit is the Magill? What fresh gas flows do you require to use for spontaneous respiration? What is the explanation for the efficiency of this circuit? What are the disadvantages of this circuit?

5. An ITU patient has become oliguric postoperatively – what are the possible causes? How would you manage this patient? How does dopamine work? What dose would you use? What happens as you increase the dose of dopamine?

6. You are called to see an obstetric patient at term who is fitting – what would you do? What is the differential diagnosis? What are the problems encountered when resuscitating an obstetric patient who has arrested? How can they be overcome?

7. Describe how an ambu bag works. How can you increase the inspired oxygen concentration? Is it possible to give 100% oxygen with an ambu bag?

Viva 23

1. How high do you require a patient's haemoglobin to be prior to anaesthesia? Do you transfuse patients overnight prior to anaesthesia? Tell me about the oxygen cascade. What is oxygen flux? What is its relevance to clinical anaesthesia?
2. What methods are there available to humidify respired gases in intensive care? What are the advantages and disadvantages of each?
3. What physiological changes take place during acute hypovolaemia? On which vessels does the sympathetic nervous system exert the most influence? Which agents would you choose to anaesthetize a hypovolaemic patient and why?
4. Which methods of pain relief are there available for labour? What is TENS and how does it work? Explain the gate theory of pain. What are the transmitters involved and where are they found?
5. How would you assess a severe chronic bronchitic for fitness for surgery? When would you consider taking blood gases? If the patient was scheduled for major bowel surgery how would you manage the anaesthetic?
6. What is the probable cause of a patient suddenly complaining of severe pain as you injected your induction agent? What would you do? How would you perform a sympathetic blockade of the patient's arm? What are the dangers of stellate ganglion block? How would you perform one?
7. What are the problems in supplying 100% oxygen via a facemask to the postoperative patient? How does a Ventimask work? What is entrainment ratio? What is the flow of oxygen used on a 40% Ventimask and what is the resulting flow at the patient's face?

Viva 24

1. What are the causes of heat loss during general anaesthesia? How can we minimize these? What adverse effects can this loss of temperature have on the patient?
2. What sort of needle do you use for peripheral nerve blocks? What are the advantages of using a short-bevelled needle? How do you use a nerve stimulator? What are the theoretical advantages in using sheathed needles? How could you provide regional anaesthesia for a meniscectomy? What are the three nerves blocked in a 'three-in-one' nerve block and what are their nerve roots?
3. What are the possible causes of chest pain in a patient within 10 days of a hip replacement? What factors increase the likelihood of a patient

developing a deep venous thrombosis in the postoperative period? What can we do to reduce the incidence, particularly in hip surgery?

4. What physiological changes occur during pregnancy? When do the peak changes take place in the cardiovascular system? What are the significant changes with respect to anaesthesia?

5. How does a rotameter work? Why is it gas specific? What are the principles involved at low and high flows? How else can you measure flow of gas?

6. What are the problems associated with dental anaesthesia and chair dentals in particular? What equipment would you have available for a list of chair dentals?

7. What methods of sedation are there for patients in intensive care? Are there any problems with using midazolam? etomidate? thiopental? propofol?

EXAMPLE VIVA ANSWER

This section has been included to give some indication of how to answer a series of viva questions and is particularly aimed at those starting their viva practice for the first time. The first important lesson is that unless the question is very simple and requires a short answer you should pause for a moment to consider fully what the examiner has asked. The pause should not be longer than 10–15 seconds even for the most searching of questions or it will lead the examiner to believe you are having problems. Use this time to consider the question, the important points you want to bring out in your answer and the structure you are going to follow.

Example 1

The examiner hands you a Bain circuit and asks *'What is this?'*

This is a short question that requires a simple answer and you should not pause before replying *'This is a Bain circuit, sir/madam'*.

The examiner can then lead on to the next question and you have scored your first point. *'What can you tell me about this circuit?'*

Now is the time to pause and consider, as the answer to this question is large. What are the important points to cover?

Important points for a piece of equipment include:

— A simple description
— A history of its development
— Advantages and disadvantages

This has now given you a structure to follow.

Description

'It is a coaxial circuit available in various lengths (2.5 and 5.0 m commonly available) which delivers the fresh gas flow down the inner tube and removes the exhaled gases down the outer.

'It is a modified type D circuit according to the Mapleson classification.

'The APL (adjustable pressure limiting valve) is situated at the proximal end of the circuit and is designed to limit the maximum pressure generated in the circuit to 60 cm of water.'

History

'It was described by two Canadian anaesthetists, Bain and Spoerel, in 1972 but a similar coaxial circuit was used in 1940s by Pask and MacIntosh during the development of the Mae West life jacket.'

Advantages and disadvantages

'The presence of the APL at the proximal end of the circuit allows easy scavenging of waste gases and transition of modes of ventilation (between spontaneous respiration and IPPV).

'The single tube is lightweight and the lack of valve at the distal end reduces the bulk of the circuit, making it suitable for head and neck surgery.

'It is very efficient in the use of fresh gases during IPPV, requiring a flow of about 80 ml/kg to maintain normocapnia and above 100 ml/kg to provide hypocapnia.

'This formula for fresh gas flow is, however, dependent on the minute ventilation of the patient being greater than the fresh gas flow.

'The relationship between the fresh gas flow and minute ventilation is shown by graphing them together and it can be seen that a series of curves (isopleths) are produced that correspond to a given level of P_aco_2. [Candidates who cannot explain this concept are recommended to read the chapter on 'Breathing systems and vaporizers' by M J Jones in *Anaesthesia*, edited by W S Nimmo and G Smith (1989).]

'This relationship means that when the fresh gas flow is set to 80 ml/kg during IPPV then the minute ventilation can be increased to large levels without causing hypocapnia – a feature that can be useful in those with chest disease.

'Disadvantages include the fact that the circuit is inefficient of fresh gas flow during spontaneous respiration, requiring a fresh gas flow of 250–300 ml/kg (2.5–3 × minute ventilation) to prevent rebreathing; however in clinical use flows nearer 100–150 ml/kg are used and rebreathing is accepted.

'The inner tube can be difficult to inspect and if it becomes dislodged at the proximal end of the circuit the patient then has a very large dead space.

'There is appreciable resistance to gas flow, increasing the work of breathing for the patient.'

At some stage during this answer the examiner may well interrupt to ask a specific question about what you have just said or to help direct your answer in the direction he/she wishes you to follow. Be prepared to answer questions about subjects you bring up, such as the 'isopleths'; in general try not to bring up subjects that you do not understand. Try and give the best answer you can avoiding anything you are unsure about. However, if asked about something you don't know then don't panic, be honest with the examiner and he/she will often help lead you into an answer or try another question. It is important to remember to consider each question and, if you do not understand what the examiner is asking, then tell him/her and ask if he/she can rephrase the question.

If the examiner moves you on to another subject quickly after you have started your answer then again do not panic. This can be a sign that the examiner is happy with your knowledge of the present topic and now wants to move on to another.

The examiner may next ask '*How would you describe sodium thiopental to a new colleague in anaesthesia?*'

This is a question that again merits a momentary pause for considering your answer. The plan you might use for any drug could be:

— A simple statement of what it is
— A description of its presentation
— Its dosage, pharmacokinetics and pharmacodynamics
— Indications and contraindications
— Problems associated with its use

Simple statement
'*It is a thiobarbiturate, being the sulphur analogue of pentobarbitone, and is used as an induction agent.*'

Description of its presentation
'*It is supplied in ampoules of yellow powder (the sodium salt) with dry nitrogen above. It also contains six parts per 100 by weight of anhydrous sodium carbonate which is added to prevent precipitation of the insoluble free acid by contamination from atmospheric CO_2. Water is added to prepare a 2.5% solution which has a pH of 10.5.*'

Dosage, pharmacokinetics and pharmacodynamics
'*It is used in a dose of 3–5 mg/kg depending on the age and condition of the patient, particularly requiring reduction in hypovolaemic patients.*

'*Its principal effects are on the CNS due to rapid uptake by richly perfused brain tissue of the non-ionized unbound fraction leading to loss of consciousness, and dose-dependent depression of the respiratory and vasomotor centres. This results in a drop in blood pressure which can be added to by a direct effect on the myocardium at higher dose levels.*

'*Emergence from a sleep dose occurs in 5–10 min and is due to redistribution of the drug. Very little is excreted unchanged by the kidney: it is metabolized by the liver – plasma clearance of 3 ml/kg/min.*'

It is unlikely that the examiner will allow you to proceed through your entire knowledge of the drug (if you cannot speak extensively about any induction agent you use regularly then you do not deserve to pass the exam). The examiner will probably ask a supplementary question to point you in a particular direction, e.g. *'How should your colleague recognize intra-arterial injection?'* These questions may be more limited in their scope and deal with something one should be familiar with and so there should be little delay in answering.

'Every patient should be asked if his or her hand is comfortable as you inject the first part of your dose of induction agent. Complaint of particularly severe pain accompanied by blanching of the hand should be treated as intra-arterial injection.'

'How would you treat this condition?'

'Firstly, stop the injection but try and keep the cannula in the vessel. Consider injecting a vasodilator directly into the vessel and heparinized saline. If the cannula is no longer present, consider performing a sympathetic blockade on the affected limb.'

'How would you perform a sympathetic blockade for the upper limb?'

Again it is time to stop and consider your answer.

'The options open to me would include performing an axillary block, a stellate ganglion block or a Bier's block using guanethidine.'

At this stage it is legitimate to say *'I have no experience in performing stellate ganglion blockade, so I would choose to use an axillary block.'* (if this applies!)

However the examiner may still proceed to ask about the theory of stellate ganglion block.

Thus the viva may chop and change, moving from one subject to another at the examiner's discretion; however it can also be seen that the candidate has some control over the direction the viva takes. Selective answering, attempting to avoid black holes in one's knowledge and placing of emphasis on techniques one has actually used can help.

Experience is the key: the candidate should use every opportunity to extend his or her knowledge but more importantly to gain practice in the various techniques used in anaesthesia and intensive care. This is true for both Part I and Part II. It is obvious to examiners when you are answering from practical experience rather than using theory gleaned from textbooks.

Core references

INTRODUCTION

In addition to establishing a sound theoretical knowledge from the study of major anaesthetic texts, candidates should be familiar with all the major anaesthetic journals. Where possible we have provided key references next to the answer plans that should be reviewed by the candidate.

A knowledge of important articles constitutes a firm basis of anaesthetic knowledge and is useful for authoritative answering of examination questions.

Review articles, postgraduate educational issues and CEPD articles appearing within the 5-year period prior to the examination are important and journals issued in the weeks prior to the oral examination are required reading. The candidate should not limit him/herself to purely anaesthetic journals and is advised to examine editorials in the *British Medical Journal* and reviews in the *New England Journal of Medicine* for relevant articles.

However, there are a number of older references that may be useful to the candidate. Some, such as the *Triennial Confidential Report on Maternal Mortality*, are required reading; others are a source of useful information not readily available in textbooks. A selection is listed on the following pages with an indication of their importance and a brief summary. It is recommended, however, that the original papers are consulted. Most should prove interesting and the journals in which they appear should be readily available in medical libraries.

PAEDIATRICS

Ayre P 1937 Anaesthesia for hare-lip and cleft palate operations on babies. British Journal of Surgery 25: 131–132
One of the first publications from Newcastle on the development of the Ayre's T-piece. Worth reading for the language alone.

Ayre P 1956 The T-piece technique. British Journal of Anaesthesia 28: 520
Description of original T-piece as described by Ayre in 1937 with a discussion of the required fresh gas flow.

Jackson Rees G 1950 Anaesthesia in the newborn. British Medical Journal 2: 1419
Review of Liverpool practice of neonatal anaesthesia with first description of 'a double ended bag to the exhaust limb of the Ayre's T-piece' – the Jackson Rees modification.

EQUIPMENT

Bain J A, Spoerel W E 1972 A streamlined anaesthetic system. Canadian Anaesthesiology Society Journal 19: 462

Bain J A, Spoerel W E 1973 Flow requirement for a modified Mapleson D system during controlled ventilation. Canadian Anaesthesiology Society Journal 20: 629
Original description of the Bain circuit and a recommendation of 70 ml/kg/min fresh gas flow during IPPV in adults to prevent hypercapnia.

George R J D, Geddes D M 1985 High frequency ventilation. British Journal of Hospital Medicine 33(6): 344–349
Simple explanation of high frequency ventilation, the principles and its clinical application.

Holmes C McK, Spears G F S 1977 Very-nearly-closed-circuit anaesthesia – a computer analysis. Anaesthesia 32: 846–851
With increasing interest in closed circuit anaesthesia this paper provides useful information about the behaviour of a circle system and the flows necessary to ensure appropriate anaesthetic agent concentrations.

Macintosh R R, Pask E A 1957 The testing of life jackets. British Journal of Industrial Medicine 14: 168–176
First report of the use of a double lumen (coaxial) circuit in anaesthesia. Used in 1943–1945 to anaesthetize a subject who was then placed in a swimming pool to test life jackets.

Macintosh R R 1943 A new laryngoscope. Lancet 1: 205
Original description of the Macintosh laryngoscope.

Mapleson W W 1954 The elimination of rebreathing in various semi-closed anaesthetic systems. British Journal of Anaesthesia 26: 323
Explanation of the theoretical fresh gas flows required for the various circuits to prevent rebreathing.

Mapleson W W 1960 The concentration of anaesthetics in closed circuits, with special reference to halothane. I. Theoretical study. British Journal of Anaesthesia 32: 298

Galloon S 1960 The concentration of anaesthetics in closed circuits, with special reference to halothane. II. Laboratory and theatre investigations. British Journal of Anaesthesia 32: 310

Mushin W W, Galloon S 1960 The concentration of anaesthetics in closed circuits, with special reference to halothane. III. Clinical aspects. British Journal of Anaesthesia 32: 324

A series of three papers from Cardiff which clarified the performance of vaporizers in (VIC) and out (VOC) of circuit in low-flow closed-circuit anaesthesia.

Newton N I, Adams A P 1978 Excessive airway pressure during anaesthesia – hazards, effects and prevention. Anaesthesia 33: 689–699
Review of potential causes and effects of barotrauma. Techniques for protecting the patient are reviewed.

Newton N I, Hillman K M, Varley J G 1981 Automatic ventilation with the Ayre's T-piece – a modification of the Nuffield Series 200 ventilator for neonatal and paediatric use. Anaesthesia 36: 22–36
Article about the development of the 'Newton valve' for the Nuffield ventilator. Contains useful review of the possible techniques of ventilating with the T-piece.

CARDIOVASCULAR SYSTEM

Cokkinos D V, Vordis E M 1976 Constancy of rate pressure product in pacing induced angina pectoris. British Heart Journal 38: 39
Suggested that the onset of ischaemia could be predicted from reference to the rate pressure product at which angina had previously occurred.

Goldman L 1983 Cardiac risks and complication of non cardiac surgery. Annals of Internal Medicine 98: 504
A description of cardiac risk factors which are weighted to give a 'Goldman Multi-factorial Risk Index'. May usefully be quoted to compare the relative risks of various cardiac findings. Of particular interest is the observation that cardiac failure was found to carry a greater risk than did recent myocardial infarction.

Loeb H S, Saudye A, Croke R P et al 1978 Effects of pharmacologically induced hypertension on myocardial ischaemia and coronary haemodynamics in patients with fixed coronary obstruction. Circulation 51: 41
Extended the rate pressure product concept by proving that tachycardia is more likely to result in ischaemia than is hypertension (increased heart rate is associated with increased O_2 demand and reduced blood flow, hypertension increases O_2 utilization but increases blood flow).

Steen P A, Tinker J H, Tarhan S 1978 Myocardial reinfarction after anaesthesia and surgery. Journal of the American Medical Association 239: 2566
Study which confirmed that there is a 30% chance of reinfarction with surgery within 3 months of an infarct, 15% between 3 months and 6 months and 5% thereafter.

INTENSIVE CARE

Conference of Medical Royal Colleges and their Faculties in the UK 1976 Diagnosis of brain death. Lancet 2: 1069 and British Medical Journal 2: 1187
Paper from the Royal College which defined brain death and established exclusions and test protocols for diagnosis.

Conference of Medical Royal Colleges and their Faculties in the UK (1979) Diagnosis of death. Lancet 1: 261 and British Medical Journal 1: 332
Further paper from the Royal Colleges extending the observations of 1976 and stating that death of the patient could be presumed to occur when 'brain death' is diagnosed (i.e. cessation of pulse and/or respiration is not required for the diagnosis of death). Both *Diagnosis of Brain Death* 1976 and *Diagnosis of Death* 1979 also appear in:

Department of Health and Social Security 1983 Cadaveric organs for transplantation – a code of practice: including the diagnosis of brain death. DHSS, London

Jennett B, Teasdale G 1977 Aspects of coma after severe head injury. Lancet 1: 878
Description of a practical system for clinical monitoring of neurological status of patients who have sustained head injury – the Glasgow Coma Scale. Three parameters are evaluated: eye opening, best motor and verbal.

Kinsella J 1993 Smoke inhalation injury – diagnosis and management. British Journal of Intensive Care 3(1): 8–14

Kulig K 1992 Initial management of ingestions of toxic substances. New England Journal of Medicine 25: 1677–1681
Short review of management of patients presenting with overdose. General management and supportive measures outlined plus useful description of how to administer the more commonly used antidotes.

OBSTETRICS

Confidential Report on Maternal Mortality 1973–1975. HMSO, London
Important conclusions relating to the deaths due to anaesthesia included:

- Antacid therapy does not adequately protect patients from the effects of acid aspiration
- Cricoid pressure is often inexpertly applied with aspiration as a consequence – skilled assistance is important
- Unrecognized oesophageal intubation is very serious; monitoring is often inadequate
- Patients died from the effects of total spinal anaesthesia after 'top-ups' for epidural anaesthesia – absence of an immediately available trained anaesthetist represents a total contraindication to epidural anaesthesia

Confidential Report on Maternal Mortality 1976–1978. HMSO, London
Important conclusions relating to the deaths due to anaesthesia included:

- Deaths due to hypoxia during failed intubation; the importance of the adoption of a 'failed intubation drill' was emphasized
- The presence of an available anaesthetist during epidural analgesia was reiterated
- Inadequate management of haemorrhage resulted in death – adoption of a policy for the management of such patients was recommended
- The difficulty of observing hypoxia in the postoperative period – observation of patients and lighting may be poor, allied to the difficulty of recognizing hypoxia

in dark-skinned patients – was emphasized. Improved postoperative care was felt necessary

Confidential Report on Maternal Mortality 1979–1981. HMSO, London
Important conclusions relating to the deaths due to anaesthesia included:

- Emphasis on importance of trained anaesthetists, assistants and facilities
- The use of two hands for cricoid pressure to maintain neck extension
- Problem of detecting cyanosis in the dark-skinned – need for special care
- Failure of postoperative care – patients should be kept in special recovery area for at least 30 min
- Suggestion that pancuronium was not suitable for obstetric practice
- Importance of having major haemorrhage protocol (example included in report)

Confidential Report on Maternal Mortality 1982–1984. HMSO, London
Last of series for England and Wales alone and contains useful overview of trends in the maternal mortality rate since 1952.
  Important conclusions relating to the deaths due to anaesthesia included:

- Emphasis on importance of experienced anaesthetist – inexperienced anaesthetists involved in most deaths
- The safety of using spontaneous breathing technique following failed intubation was pointed out
- Questioned safety and effectiveness of particulate antacids
- Trained assistant and the use of two hands for cricoid pressure again emphasized

Confidential Report on Maternal Mortality 1985–1987. HMSO, London
First combined report for the whole of the UK.
  Important conclusions relating to the deaths due to anaesthesia included:

- Requirement for monitoring (including capnography and pulse oximetry) anywhere in maternity unit where anaesthesia may be given; each unit must take measures to confirm correct placement of endotracheal tube
- Units must have a failed intubation drill
- Anaesthetist should be involved early in the management of cases of severe pre-eclampsia even if no operative delivery is planned
- All maternity units where anaesthesia is regularly given should have a recovery area facility where high-dependency care should be available
- Invasive cardiovascular monitoring should be used where indicated
- Early discussion between the obstetricians and anaesthetists about possible high-risk patients is recommended
- Availability of consultant anaesthetists, skilled assistants and monitoring equipment must be ensured

Confidential Report on Maternal Mortality 1988–1990. HMSO, London
Important conclusions relating to the deaths due to anaesthesia included:

- Capnography should be available in all areas where general anaesthesia is administered
- H_2 receptor blocking drugs should be administered to all patients who may require anaesthesia, and patients with pre-eclampsia
- Important to insert large bore cannulae and a CVP line and to call for senior anaesthetic and obstetric assistance as soon as severe blood loss is observed

- Midwifery staff looking after postoperative patients should be specifically trained in monitoring, care of the airway and resuscitative procedures and be supervised by a defined anaesthetist at all times
- Use of pulse oximetry during anaesthesia and the early postoperative period should be routine
- Adequate consultant supervision is important for maternity services

Confidential Report on Maternal Mortality 1991–1993. HMSO, London
Important conclusions relating to the deaths due to anaesthesia included:

- Still problems with airway, aspiration and hypovolaemic shock
- All obstetric patients requiring anaesthesia should be regarded as high risk. Staffing and management should reflect this
- Lack of consultant involvement is a recurring problem which must be solved
- Failure to use appropriate monitoring (especially pulse oximetry) still a problem
- First report where the requirement for intensive care was considered – importance of availability and use of intensive care where needed was stressed
- Co-operation between specialties and early involvement of consultant colleagues is vital to produce a good outcome

Confidential Report on Maternal Mortality 1994–1996. HMSO, London

- Increase in deaths due to thromboembolism, amniotic fluid embolism and sepsis
- Reduction in deaths due to haemorrhage and pregnancy induced hypertension

Reduced number of deaths directly attributed to anaesthesia but problems highlighted by the indirect deaths include:

- Continuing problem with cardiac disease
- Increasing problem with epilepsy
- Need to continue developing and updating guidelines and use regular 'Fire Drills' to practice them

Crawford J S 1985 Some maternal complications of epidural analgesia for labour. Anaesthesia 40: 1219–1225
Review of maternal complications occurring in a series of 27 000 lumbar epidural blocks administered for labour which included 100 000 top-ups by midwives. Despite the occurrence of nine potentially life-threatening complications the adherence to established protocols led to a successful outcome. This review supports that an organized epidural service provides a high level of safety for the mother.

Cunningham F G, Lindheimer M D 1992 Hypertension in pregnancy. New England Journal of Medicine 14: 927–932
Review of hypertensive disease in pregnancy covering detection, pathophysiology, prevention and management. Good review that includes differences in European and American management.

Holmes F 1960 The supine hypotensive syndrome. Its importance to the anaesthetist. Anaesthesia 15(3): 298–306
First publication in an anaesthetic journal describing aortocaval compression and its importance in both spinal and general anaesthesia in women in late pregnancy.

Mendelson C L 1946 The aspiration of stomach contents into the lungs during obstetric anaesthesia. Journal of Obstetrics and Gynecology 52: 191

First description of the aspiration syndrome which bears the author's name. 66 cases were reported and two deaths occurred due to suffocation from complete airway obstruction by solid undigested food (both patients had recently eaten). None of the remaining patients who went on to develop the aspiration syndrome died. It has been suggested that the practice of feeding these patients may have buffered their gastric acid, with consequent reduction of damage on aspiration. Other possibilities include that modern therapy has made the syndrome more dangerous; e.g. ergometrine administration has been suggested as a potential exacerbator.

Tunstall M E 1976 Failed intubation. Anaesthesia 31: 850
Extract from the Obstetric Anaesthetists' Association (OAA) meeting of March 1976 with description of the 'failed intubation drill' as practised in Aberdeen.

REGIONAL TECHNIQUES

Dripps R D, Vandam L D 1954 Long term follow up of patients who received 10 098 spinal anaesthetics: failure to discover major neurological sequelae. Journal of the American Medical Association 156: 1486

Hart J R, Whitacre R J 1951 Pencil-point needle in prevention of postspinal headache. Journal of the American Medical Association 147: 657–658
Recognition of headache following spinal anaesthesia leading to the development of the Whitacre needle.

Kenedy F, Effron A S, Perry G 1950 Grave spinal cord paralysis caused by spinal anaesthesia. Surgery, Gynecology and Obstetrics 91: 385
A damning paper from Foster Kenedy, a leading neurologist practising in America. Set the scene for the decline in popularity of spinal anaesthesia.

Moore D C, Bridenbaugh L D 1966 Spinal (subarachnoid) block. A review of 11 574 cases. Journal of the American Medical Association 195: 907
Both extensive surveys failed to reveal cases of serious neurological complications following spinal anaesthesia.

Trotter M 1947 Variations of the sacral canal: their significance in the administration of caudal analgesia. Anesthesia and Analgesia 26: 192
A large survey of sacral anatomy which highlighted the wide range of anatomical variation of the adult sacrum.

PHYSIOLOGY

Katz R L 1967 Neuromuscular effects of d-tubocurarine, edrophonium and neostigmine in man. Anaesthesiology 28: 327
Documented a wide variation in sensitivity to d-tubocurarine (0.1 mg/kg), total relaxation occurring in 7% of patients and no depression of twitch height at all in 6% of patients (supports the concept of neuromuscular monitoring).

AUDIT OF PRACTICE

Lunn J N, Mushin W W 1982 Mortality associated with anaesthesia. Nuffield Provincial Hospitals Trust, London
Report of a large survey of anaesthesia in five regions over 12 months. Important conclusions included: in 1 : 10 000 anaesthetics, death totally attributable to anaesthesia; monitoring should be more frequently employed; spinal anaesthesia can be disastrous when applied to sick patients with untreated hypovolaemia; consultation between surgeons and anaesthetists is inadequate; recovery facilities are often inadequate.

Buck N, Devlin H B, Lunn J N 1987 The report of a confidential enquiry into perioperative deaths. Nuffield Provincial Hospitals Trust/King's Fund, London
First UK enquiry to combine both anaesthetic and surgical assessment of mortality following surgery. Report concerns deaths within 30 days of an operation in three regions during 1986. Revealed that overall mortality rate was low (0.7%); the vast majority of these were elderly patients and death was unavoidable due to progression of the presenting condition. The incidence of deaths solely attributable to errors in anaesthesia was 1 : 185 000, those solely attributable to errors in surgery was 1 : 2500 and those attributable to a combination of errors in both anaesthesia and surgery was 1 : 1300. Areas of substandard care included:

- Junior staff were undertaking surgery for which they were not yet trained
- Consultant supervision was often inadequate
- Surgeons were operating outside their specialized field
- Unnecessary surgery on moribund or terminally ill patients

Report revealed lack of visiting of patients preoperatively, lack of use of monitoring equipment and lack of recovery rooms, particularly 'out of hours'.

Each subsequent NCEPOD report should be read and particular attention paid to the report summaries and any anaesthetic recommendations. The NCEPOD website at *www.ncepod.org.uk* contains all the information required.

Derrington M C, Smith G 1987 A review of studies of anaesthetic risk, morbidity and mortality. British Journal of Anaesthesia 59: 815–833

Dundee J W, McIlroy P D A 1982 The history of the barbiturates. Anaesthesia 37: 726–734

Halsey M J 1991 Occupational health and pollution from anaesthetics. A report of a seminar. Anaesthesia 46: 486–488

Imrie M M, Hall G M 1990 Body temperature and anaesthesia. British Journal of Anaesthesia 64: 346–354

Mason R A, Steane P A 1976 Carcinoid syndrome: its relevance to the anaesthetist. Anaesthesia 31: 228–242

Milledge J S, Nunn J F 1975 Criteria for fitness for anaesthesia in patients with chronic obstructive lung disease. British Medical Journal 3: 670
Described three groups of patients where $FEV_1 < 1$ litre or <50% and predicted that they were likely to experience differing postoperative courses:

Group I	Pco_2 normal, Po_2 normal – generally uncomplicated
Group II	Pco_2 normal, Po_2 reduced – require prolonged postoperative O_2 therapy
Group III	Pco_2 raised, Po_2 reduced – likely to require postoperative mechanical ventilation

Nimmo W S 1984 Effect of anaesthesia on gastric motility and emptying. British Journal of Anaesthesia 56: 29

Reynolds F 1987 Adverse effects of local anaesthetics. British Journal of Anaesthesia 59: 78–95

Saddler J M, Horsey P J 1987 The new generation gelatins. A review of their history, manufacture and properties. Anaesthesia 42: 998–1004

Sellick R A 1961 Cricoid pressure to control regurgitation of stomach contents during induction of anaesthesia: preliminary communication. Lancet 2: 404
First description of 'Sellick's manoeuvre'. Studies of the oesophageal pressure were included.

Smith G, Cotton B R 1984 The lower oesophageal sphincter and anaesthesia. British Journal of Anaesthesia 56: 37

Thromboemboli Risk Factors (THRIFT) Consensus Group 1992 Risk of and prophylaxis for venous thromboembolism in hospital patients. British Medical Journal 305: 567–574

Trunkey D 1991 Initial treatment of patients with extensive trauma. New England Journal of Medicine 18: 1259–1263

Vaughan R S, Lunn J N 1973 Potassium and the anaesthetist. Anaesthesia 28: 118–131

Wells D G, Bjorksten A R 1989 Monoamine oxidase inhibitors revisited. Canadian Journal of Anaesthesia 36: 64–74

Whitwam J G 1977 APUD cells and the apudomas – a concept relevant to anaesthesia and endocrinology. Anaesthesia 32: 879–888

Williamson L M, Lowe S, Love E M et al 1999 Serious hazards of transfusion (SHOT) initiative: analysis of the first two annual reports British Medical Journal 319: 16–19

Glossary of useful terms

This section includes many little facts and figures that may be of use to the examination candidate. The management regimes for anaphylaxis and malignant hyperpyrexia plus the machine checklist based on the guidelines produced by the Association of Anaesthetists are included. It can be used both as a revision aid and to help candidates practise answering viva questions with each other. The technique of developing a collection of small notes about key topics in anaesthesia can be very useful as part of the revision process and is particularly helpful in the last few days leading up to the exam.

ACETYLCHOLINE
$CH_3—CO—OCH_2—CH_2—N(CH_3)_3$

- Synthesized from choline and acetyl coenzyme A in axoplasm of cholinergic nerve terminals catalysed by enzyme choline acetyltransferase
- The enzyme is synthesized in the ribosomes in the cell bodies and passes to the nerve terminals where its concentration is highest
- Activity is increased by treatment with prednisolone and other glucocorticoids (explains beneficial effect in myasthenia)
- Most of choline comes from diet, acetylco A is synthesized from pyruvate

ACh storage

- 1% of vesicles at nerve terminal form the 'readily releasable store' responsible for the maintenance of transmitter release under low activity
- 80% is in 'releasable store'
- Remainder in 'stationary store'
- Axon terminals have spherical vesicles that are made in the cell body and pass down by axoplasmic flow. 80% of ACh is contained in these, the rest is in cytosol

- Active transport system exists to transport ACh into vesicles

ADHESION
- Attraction between molecules of two different substances (cf. COHESION)

ADIABETIC
- Changes of state in a gas; occurs when allowing gas to expand or be compressed without allowing the gas to exchange heat energy with its surroundings, e.g. cryoprobe

ADRENALINE (EPINEPHRINE) (see also catecholamine)
Maximum dose allowable depends on condition of patient and reason for use. As part of local anaesthesia or if administered separately to reduce surgical bleeding consider 3 µg/kg.

ADULT RESPIRATORY DISTRESS SYNDROME (ARDS)
- First described in 1967 in *The Lancet* (by Ashbaugh, Bigelow, Petty & Levine) in 12 patients:
    — X-ray evidence of patchy alveolar infiltration
    — reduced lung compliance
    — refractory hypoxaemia
    — PM findings of hyaline membranes and microscopic atelectasis
- Concept of varying disease severity was recognized with consensus definition in 1994
- **Acute lung injury** recognised as an entity and ARDS defined as its most severe manifestation
- Survivors usually have little pulmonary dysfunction
- Mortality appears to be decreasing (down from 68% to 36%), particularly in younger patients and those with sepsis
- Improvements linked to:
    — acceptance of lower targets for oxygenation and CO_2 clearance
    — protective ventilation strategies which increase mean airway pressure – pressure limited inverse ratio ventilation and higher levels of PEEP, prone ventilation
    — general improvements in supportive care, as most die from associated systems failure or multiple organ system failure

AIRWAY RESISTANCE
- 80% of total airway resistance is generated in the larger airways down to 2 mm diameter – flow here is laminar in normal quiet respiration
- When flow increases (exercise, respiratory distress) laminar flow is replaced with turbulence, greatly increasing the work of breathing

ALBUMIN
- Most abundant plasma protein, accounts for 55–60% of serum protein
- Single polypeptide chain of 585 amino acids arranged in series of alpha helices folded and held by 17 disulphide bridges
- Molecular weight 66 500 daltons

- Total albumin pool is 3.5–5.0 g/kg (250–300 g in average adult)
- 42% in plasma, rest in extravascular compartments
- Synthesis in liver 194 mg/kg/day and this can increase 2.0–2.7 times
- Provides 80% of the colloid oncotic pressure (COP) of 25 mmHg

ALFENTANIL

- Analogue of fentanyl with 10–20% of its potency and shorter duration of action

ALLERGY penicillin

- 1–10% of population affected
- Anaphylactic reactions in 15–40/100 000 treated patients
- Fatal outcome in 1.5–2/100 000 treated patients
- Patient with specific history of allergy to penicillin is at least six times more likely to develop a reaction than a non-allergic patient on subsequent exposure

ALLIGATION – VENTURI MASKS

This allows calculation of the entrainment ratio
A is % of oxygen supplied to mask (100%), B is % of oxygen in atmosphere (make 20% for ease of calculation), C is the concentration the mask is calibrated for (40% in this case)

$$
\begin{array}{ccccc}
A \searrow & \nearrow C\text{-}B & 100 & 20 & \\
& C & & 40 & 20/60 = \text{entrainment ratio } ^1/_3 \\
B \nearrow & \searrow A\text{-}C & 20 & 60 &
\end{array}
$$

so at 8 l 100% O_2 entrains 24 l of air, so resultant flow = 32 l

ALVEOLAR GAS EQUATION

$$P_{AO_2} = Pio_2 - (P_{A}co_2/R) + F$$

where $F = P_{A}co_2 \times Fio_2 \times (1-R)/R$

AMETOP

Tetracaine (amethocaine) 4%, Xantan gum, methyl and propyl-p hydroxy-benzoate, water and saline

ANAPHYLACTIC REACTION

- Hypersensitivity (type 1) reaction to allergen to which patient has been exposed earlier, results from Ag/Ab interaction

ANAPHYLACTOID REACTION

- Similar picture but no Ag/Ab interaction; results from direct influence on mast cells

ANAPHYLAXIS TREATMENT

- Stop administration of drug(s) likely to have caused the anaphylaxis
- Maintain airway; give 100% oxygen
- Lie patient flat with feet elevated
- Give adrenaline (epinephrine). This may be given intramuscularly in a dose of 0.5–1 mg (0.5–1 ml of 1:1000) and may be repeated every

10 min according to the arterial pressure and pulse until improvement occurs

Alternatively, 50–100 μg intravenously over 1 min has been recommended (0.5–1 ml of 1 : 10 000) for hypotension with titration of further doses as required

In a patient with cardiovascular collapse, 0.5–1 mg (5–10 ml of 1 : 10 000) may be required intravenously in divided doses by titration. This should be given at a rate of 0.1 mg/min stopping when a response has been obtained

- Start intravascular volume expansion with crystalloid or colloid

Secondary therapy
- Antihistamines – chlorphenamine (chlorpheniramine) 10–20 mg by slow intravenous infusion
- Corticosteroids – 100–300 mg hydrocortisone IV
- Catecholamine infusions – starting doses: adrenaline (epinephrine) 4–8 μg/min [0.05–0.1 μg/kg/min]; noradrenaline (norepinephrine) 4–8 μg/min [0.05–0.1 μg/kg/min]; isoprenaline 0.05–1 μg/min
- Consider bicarbonate (0.5–1.0 mmol/kg IV) for acidosis
- Airway evaluation (before extubation)
- Bronchodilators may be required for persistent bronchospasm

ANTIDEPRESSANTS
Monoamine oxidase inhibitors (MAOIs)
- Act by forming stable complex with monoamine oxidase, hence need to be discontinued for 10–14 days for sufficient new enzyme production
- Result in build up of noradrenaline (norepinephrine), 5-HT and dopamine
- Dangers with interactions with sympathomimetics, certain opioids
- Delay of routine surgery has been recommended but must remember dangers of depression

Selective serotonin reuptake inhibitors (SSRIs), e.g. fluoxetine (Prozac), sertraline (Zoloft)
- Preoperatively
  — ensure not hyponatraemic due to inappropriate ADH secretion (especially in elderly)
  — may impair platelet aggregation ? bleeding time
  — stopping them may cause withdrawal syndrome
- Interactions
  — midazolam metabolism may be inhibited
  — serotomimetic drugs (pethidine, pentazocine) may predispose patient to serotonin syndrome (see SEROTONIN SYNDROME)

APNOEIC OXYGENATION
- rate of rise $P_a\text{CO}_2$ = 0.4 kPa/min

ASA STATUS

Grade 1
Patient has no organic, physiological, biochemical or psychiatric disturbance. The pathological process for which operation is to be performed is localized and does not entail a systemic disturbance

Grade 2
Mild to moderate systemic disturbance caused either by the condition to be treated surgically or by other pathophysiological processes, e.g. slight heart disease, mild diabetes, hypertension or anaemia, extreme obesity, chronic bronchitis

Grade 3
Severe systemic disturbance or disease from whatever cause, even though it may not be possible to define the degree of disability with finality, e.g. severe limiting organic heart disease, severe diabetes, angina, healed MI

Grade 4
Severe systemic disorders that are already life-threatening, not always correctable by operation, e.g. heart disease showing marked signs of failure

Grade 5
The moribund patient who has little chance of survival but is submitted to operation in desperation, e.g. burst aneurysm, major cerebral trauma with increase in ICP, massive pulmonary embolus

ASPIRATION

Incidence
- 0.031%–0.047% for routine GA
- 0.11% for emergency general surgery
- 0.15–0.22% for caesarean section

AVOGADRO'S HYPOTHESIS
- Equal volumes of gases at the same temperature and pressure contain equal numbers of molecules

AZEOTROPES
- A mixture which vaporizes in the same proportions as the volume concentrations of the components in solution, e.g. ether : halothane 1 : 2

BLOOD GROUPS

Group	Antigen on RBC	Antibodies in serum	Frequency %
O	None	Anti A and B	47
A	A	Anti B	42
B	B	Anti A	8
AB	A and B	None	3

O universal donor.
AB universal recipient.

Rhesus

- Contains at least five important antigens of which D is most important
  + ve   85%
  − ve   15%
  controlled by three pairs of allelomorphic genes occupying three
  separate but closely linked loci on each pair of chromosomes
  C and its allele c
  E and its allele e
  D and its allele d
  Rhesus negative is taken to mean absence of D antigen in recipients but
  for donors must be cde/cde

BETA BLOCKERS

Intrinsic sympathomimetic activity	Membrane stabilizing activity	β_1 Selectivity
Oxprenolol	Propranolol	Atenolol
Practolol	Oxprenolol	Practolol
	Acebutolol	Acebutolol

Lipophylic
Propranolol, metoprolol, acebutolol, oxprenolol

Water-soluble
Atenolol, nadolol, sotalol

BOYLES MACHINE
- Working pressure 4 bar = 400 kPa
- Machine pressure relief valve 34 kPa = 350 cm/water
- Oxygen bypass ≥ 35 l/min

Machine checklist
The trainee should check the machine before each list using the current
guidelines published by the Association of Anaesthetists, as follows:
    Check that the anaesthetic machine is connected to the electricity supply
(if appropriate) and switched on.
    Check that an oxygen analyser is present on the anaesthetic machine.

- Ensure that the analyser is switched on, checked and calibrated
- The oxygen sensor should be placed where it can monitor the
  composition of the gases leaving the common gas outlet

Identify and take note of the gases that are being supplied by pipeline, con-
firming with a 'tug-test' that each pipeline is correctly inserted into the
appropriate gas supply terminal.
    Note: Carbon dioxide cylinders should not be present on the anaesthetic
machine unless requested by the anaesthetist. A blanking plug should be
fitted to any empty cylinder yoke.

- Check that the anaesthetic machine is connected to a supply of oxygen and that an adequate supply of oxygen is available from a reserve oxygen cylinder
- Check that adequate supplies of other gases (nitrous oxide, air) are available and connected as appropriate
- Check that all pipeline pressure gauges in use on the anaesthetic machine indicate 400 kPa.

Check the operation of flowmeters.

- Ensure that each flow control valve operates smoothly and that the bobbin moves freely throughout its range
- Check the operation of the emergency oxygen bypass control

Check the vaporizer(s).

- Ensure that each vaporizer is adequately, but not over-filled
- Ensure that each vaporizer is correctly seated on the back bar and not tilted
- Check the vaporizer for leaks (with vaporizer on and off) by temporarily occluding the common gas outlet
- When checks have been completed turn the vaporizer(s) off
- A leak test should be performed immediately after changing any vaporizer

Check the breathing system to be employed.

- The system should be visually inspected for correct configuration. All connections should be secured by 'push and twist'
- A pressure leak test should be performed on the breathing system by occluding the patient port and compressing the reservoir bag
- The correct operation of unidirectional valves should be carefully checked

Check that the ventilator is configured appropriately for its intended use.

- Ensure that the ventilator tubing is correctly configured and securely attached
- Set the controls for use and ensure that an adequate pressure is generated during the inspiratory phase
- Check that the pressure relief valve functions
- Check that the disconnect alarm functions correctly
- Ensure that an alternative means to ventilate the patient's lungs is available

Check that the anaesthetic gas scavenging system is switched on and is functioning correctly.

- Ensure that the tubing is attached to the appropriate expiratory port(s) of the breathing system or ventilator

Check that all ancillary equipment that may be needed is present and working.

- This includes laryngoscopes, intubation aids, intubation forceps, bougies, etc. and appropriately sized facemasks, airways, tracheal tubes and connectors
- Check that the suction apparatus is functioning and that all connections are secure
- Check that the patient can be tilted head-down on the trolley, operating table or bed

Ensure that the appropriate monitoring equipment is present, switched on and calibrated ready for use.

- Set all default alarm limits as appropriate (it may be necessary to place the monitors in the stand-by mode to avoid unnecessary alarms before being connected to the patient)

BUNSEN SOLUBILITY COEFFICIENT

- Volume of gas, corrected to s.t.p., which dissolves in one unit volume of the liquid at the temperature concerned, where the partial pressure of the gas above the liquid is one standard atmosphere

BUPIVACAINE

- Chiral compound, racemic mixture (50:50) of two enantiomers due to single asymmetric carbon atom
- Suggestion that bulk of CNS and cardiovascular toxicity comes with dextro or R (+) isomer.
- Levo or S(−) has less inherent toxicity; preclinical trials suggest LD50 that is 1.2–3.3 times higher and convulsion threshold 1.7 times higher
- pH = 5.5 or 3.9 with adrenaline (epinephrine)
- Max dose 2 mg/kg in any 4 h period
- developed 1960s
- toxicity:
  — 1.6–2.0 μg/ml – mild signs
  — 2.3–5.0 μg/ml – more severe signs
- Albright's editorial in *Anesthesiology* (1979; 51: 285) first drew attention to cardiotoxicity
- It binds to cardiac Na channels and is only slowly removed. This produces slowing of conduction (manifests as prolonged PR and QRS intervals) predisposing to re-entrant arrhythmias

CALORIE

- Is the amount of energy required to raise temperature of 1 kg of water by 1°C
- calorie = 4.18 joules
- kilocalorie or Calorie = 4.18 kilojoules

Carbohydrate	4.1 Calories per g
Fat	9.3 Calories per g
Protein	4.1 Calories per g

CARRIAGE OF GASES IN BLOOD
Oxygen
Solution

$$0.003\,\text{ml}/\text{mmHg}/100\,\text{ml} = 0.3\,\text{ml}/100\,\text{ml}/100\,\text{mmHg}\ (13\,\text{kPa})$$
$$= 0.01\,\text{mmol}/\text{l}/\text{kPa}$$

Haemoglobin

$$1.34\ \text{or}\ 1.39\,\text{ml}/\text{g} = 0.06\,\text{mmol}/\text{l}$$

Carbon dioxide

	Arterial	Venous
Solution	3	3.4
Haemoglobin	3	3.7
Bicarbonate	42	44.9
TOTALS	48	52

CATECHOLAMINE

	CH_3
amino	NH
alpha carbon	CH_2
beta carbon	CHOH

OH on carbons 3 and 4 (4 is at bottom of catechol ring)

Structure-activity relationship
- Directly acting drugs have two OH groups on C3,4 – adrenaline (epinephrine), NA, dopamine
- Indirectly acting drugs have either no or only one OH group on C3,4 – ephedrine, tyramine, and metaraminol

Note
- OH on beta carbon necessary for direct action
- CH_3 on the alpha carbon prevents metabolism by MAO – ephedrine, metaraminol
- Substitution with larger groups on the amino position enhances beta activity – salbutamol, terbutaline, and isoprenaline

CENTRAL NERVOUS SYSTEM
Cerebral perfusion pressure (CPP)
CPP = MAP – ICP
Normal CPP = 80 mmHg
Critical CPP = 30 mmHg
Auto regulation (MAP 60–180 mmHg)
$P_a co_2$
If reduce to 3.5 kPa → **reduce** cerebral blood flow by 30%
If increase to 8–11 kPa → **increase** by 100%

Blood flow
50 ml/min/100 g equates to about 750 ml/min
Critical flow = 18–24 ml per 100 g/min

CISATRACURIUM
- Benzylisoquinoliniums
- Cisatracurium besylate is one of 10 stereoisomers in atracurium (about 15%)
- Similar profile to atracurium but less histamine release

CLARK ELECTRODE (POLAROGRAPHIC ELECTRODE)
Platinum cathode and silver/silver chloride anode bathed in potassium chloride electrolyte.
Uses battery and meter to detect current.
Oxygen dissolving in electrolyte reacts at cathode to provide current proportional to oxygen concentration.

COANDA EFFECT
- Wall attachment described in 1932 by Coanda (Romanian)

COCAINE
- Maximum dose 1.5–3.0 mg/kg (up to 200 mg)

CODEINE (methylmorphine)
- Semisynthetic opioid produced by substitution of a methyl group for the hydroxyl group on carbon 3
- 10% demethylated to morphine in the liver (but enzyme responsible deficient in 7% of caucasians)
- Remainder demethylated to norcodeine, which is inactive

COHESION
- Mutual attraction between molecules of a substance

CONCENTRATION EFFECT
- Higher the inspired concentration, the more rapid is the alveolar rate of rise toward the inspired concentration

CONCENTRATIONS

1%	1 in 100	10 mg/ml (i.e. 1 g in 100 ml of solvent)
0.1%	1 in 1000	1 mg/ml
0.01%	1 in 10 000	0.1 mg/ml
0.001%	1 in 100 000	0.01 mg/ml
0.0005%	1 in 200 000	0.005 mg/ml

CRITICAL PRESSURE
- The pressure (i.e. vapour pressure) of a substance at its critical temperature

CRITICAL TEMPERATURE
- The temperature above which a substance cannot be liquefied, however much pressure is applied

CYLINDERS
- Molybdenum steel
- Oxygen, Entonox, air and helium stored as a gas
- Nitrous oxide, carbon dioxide and cyclopropane as a liquid
- Valve block shows weight of empty cylinder, symbol of contents and pressure of hydraulic testing
- Filling ratio (usually 0.75)

Weight of substance cylinder is filled with divided by the weight of water it could hold

DALTON'S LAW of partial pressures
- In a mixture of gases the pressure exerted by each gas is the same as that which it would exert if it alone occupied the container

DAMPING
- Dissipation of energy within an oscillating system
- The rate of dissipation of this energy must be correctly chosen by adjustment of the resistance of the system

$$\text{Damping} = \frac{\text{Viscous resistance}}{2 \times \sqrt{(\text{mass} \times \text{stiffness})}}$$

- Critical damping = where there is just no overshoot
- Optimum damping = only 7% overshoot = 64% of critical
  When used the amplitude of the recorded oscillation remains within 2% of the input signal up to two-thirds that of the undamped natural frequency

Undamped natural frequency (f_o) = $1/2\Pi$ (stiffness/mass)
In catheter transducer system (f_o) = $1/2\Pi$ (Π, $r^2 \times$ stiffness/length)

DERMATOME LANDMARKS
- C7 – middle finger
- T3 – apex axilla
- T7 – tip of xiphoid
- T10 – umbilicus
- T12 – inguinal ligament
- L3 – knee, anterior aspect
- L4 – calf, medial aspect
- L5 – calf, lateral aspect
- S1 – foot, lateral aspect
- S2 – knee, posterior aspect

DEXMEDETOMIDINE
- Imidazole derivative – highly selective, specific α_2 agonist
- Selectivity ratio 1620:1 compared to 220:1 for clonidine
- Is the dextro-stereoisomer and pharmacologically active component of medetomidine (used in veterinary practice)

- Causes a dose-dependent decrease in arterial blood pressure and heart rate associated with a decrease in serum noradrenaline (norepinephrine) concentrations
- Reduces MAC by 90% in animals, acts by stimulation of central postsynaptic alpha$_2$ receptors
- Reported to attenuate haemodynamic responses to intubation, reduce plasma concentrations of catecholamines during anaesthesia and reduce perioperative requirements for opioids

DIAMORPHINE (example of prodrug)
- Semisynthetic opioid produced by acetylation of morphine
- Deacetylated rapidly in plasma to 6-monoacetyl morphine(6-MAM) by plasma cholinesterase with a half-life of 3 minutes. 6-MAM is relatively fat-soluble and enters the CNS where it is probably further deacetylated to morphine

DIFFUSION
Graham's law
  Rate of diffusion of a gas is inversely proportional to the square root of its molecular weight.
Fick's law
  Rate of diffusion of a substance across unit area is directly proportional to the concentration gradient.

DRUG METABOLISM
- Drugs are commonly metabolized in the liver in two phases:
  Phase I – *Oxidation*: major enzyme system cytochrome P450 [CYP] (a family of haemoproteins)
  Phase II – *Conjugation*: propofol mostly metabolized by this
- CYP3A4 is of interest as it metabolizes midazolam, lidocaine (lignocaine), alfentanil, erythromycin

ELECTRICITY
- Current ampere (**A**)
  — flow of 6.24×10^{18} electrons per second (see SI units)
- Potential difference volt (**V**)
  — the potential difference which produces current of 1 ampere in a substance when the rate of energy dissipation is 1 watt
- Resistance (ohm, Ω)
  — resistance which will allow 1 ampere of current to flow with a potential difference of 1 volt
- Charge (coulomb, **C**, **Q**)
  — quantity of electrical charge which passes some point when a current of 1 ampere flows for a period of 1 second

EMLA
- Eutectic mixture of local anaesthetics (developed 1981, available UK 1986)

- Lidocaine (lignocaine) 2.5%, prilocaine 2.5%, arlatone (emulsifier), carbopol (thickener) distilled water and sodium hydroxide
- When mix crystalline bases of lidocaine (lignocaine) and prilocaine they become an oily fluid at room temperature as a result of the lowering of their respective boiling points. Mixture provides 80% active local anaesthetic in each droplet compared to 20% if lignocaine was emulsified alone

ENERGY
- Work is done or energy expended whenever the point of application of a force moves in the direction of the force
- SI unit = joule (J)

ENOXIMONE
- Selective phosphodiesterase inhibitor
- Significant inotropic and vasodilator properties
- Additive to dobutamine

ENTRAINMENT RATIO
- Entrained flow divided by driving flow

EPINEPHRINE *see* ADRENALINE

EXPONENTIAL PROCESS
- Rate of change of a quantity at any time is proportional to the quantity at that time

Exponential formula

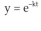

$y = e^{-kt}$

air flow on expiration

$y = e^{kt}$

bacterial growth

$y = 1-e^{-kt}$

flow into lungs with contant pressure generator

$y = 1-e^{kt}$

$y = x^2$ (2 = exponent and is fixed in this case)
$y = k^x$ (x is a variable exponent)
    in medicine normally find exponential process as described above –
    natural exponential function and constant $k = 2.7183 = e$

EQUIPMENT
- Class I   earthed casing
- Class II   double insulated, no earth required
- Internally powered   built in power source, usually batteries

FENTANYL
- Synthetic opioid derived from phenylpiperidines
- Potency 50–100 that of morphine
- Metabolized by dealkylation to norfentanyl but also hydroxylation by cytochrome P-450

FICK PRINCIPLE
- The size of a stream may be readily calculated if we know the amount of substance which enters or leaves the stream and the concentration difference resulting from such entry or removal
- Blood flow to organ =

$$\frac{\text{rate of arrival or departure of substance}}{\text{difference in concentration of substance in arterial and venous systems}}$$

- Example in lungs
Rebreathe through spirometer and soda lime canister, if measure oxygen uptake of 250 ml/min
    Measure oxygen content, if arterial 200 ml/l and venous 150 ml/l
then flow to lungs = 250/(200 − 150) = 250/50 = 5 l/min

FLOW OF GASES
Laminar (Hagen-Poiseuille equation)

$$\text{Flow} = \frac{\pi \Delta \, Pr^4}{8\eta l}$$

where ΔP = pressure difference, r = radius of tube
   η = viscosity and l = length of tube
resistance constant as long as flow laminar

Turbulent

$$\text{Flow} = \frac{\sqrt{P(r^2)}}{lP}$$

where ρ = density
resistance alters with increasing flow rate

Orifice

$$\text{Flow} = \frac{\sqrt{P}(r^2)}{\sqrt{P}}$$

FUEL CELL
Gold cathode and lead anode bathed in potassium hydroxide electrolyte does not require battery, but uses meter to detect current.

Oxygen dissolving in electrolyte reacts at gold cathode to provide current proportional to oxygen concentration.

GABA (gamma aminobutyric acid)
• Inhibitory neurotransmitter, found in large amounts in the hippocampus, cerebellum, hypothalamus and cerebral cortex
• Subdivided into two subtypes: GABA-A and GABA-B. GABA-A responsible for sedation and anxiolysis; other subtype has unknown function
• Receptor controls chloride channel
• Benzodiazepines influence these receptors by acting on benzodiazepine receptors, which form complexes with GABA receptors

GAS
• Substance above its critical temperature (cf. VAPOUR)

GAS LAWS
• Boyle's law
    At constant temperature volume varies inversely with pressure ($V \propto 1/P$)
• Charles law (Gay Lussac's law)
    At constant pressure volume varies directly with absolute temperature ($V \propto T$)
• Third perfect gas law
    At constant volume pressure varies directly with absolute temperature ($P \propto T$)
• See also Universal gas constant

HAEMACCEL
• Cross-linked gelatin prepared from collagen in animal tissue
• Average molecular weight 35 000

HEAT
• Heat capacity
    The amount of heat required to raise the temperature of a given object by 1 kelvin
• Specific heat capacity
    The amount of heat required to raise the temperature of 1 kg of substance by 1 kelvin

- Specific latent heat

    The amount of heat required to convert 1 kg of a substance from one phase to another at a given temperature

HENDERSON–HASSELBALCH EQUATION

$$pH = pK_a + \log(A^-/HA) \text{ or } pH = pK_a + \log(HCO_3^-/H_2CO_3)$$

HEPARIN

- Unfractionated heparin (UFH) is a heterogeneous mixture of polysaccharides with an average molecular weight of 15000 daltons

Low molecular weight heparins (LMWH)

- Prepared by chemical or enzymatic depolymerization of UFH; those used in UK have mean molecular weights in range 4–6000 daltons
- Are weaker inhibitors of thrombin (factor IIa) than UFH but inhibit the coagulation enzyme Xa to a similar degree. The ratio of anti-Xa to anti-IIa activity is therefore 2–4 times higher than that of UFH. Anti-Xa activity appears to be the major (but not sole) determinant of its anticoagulant activity
- Better absorbed than UFH and bind less to proteins in plasma and in the endothelial wall
- Bioavailability is around 90% at all doses (10–30% for UFH)
- $t_{1/2}$ is 4 h (UFH 1.5 h) sufficient to provide anticoagulant action with once-daily injection
- UFH partly metabolized in the liver and partly eliminated by the kidneys
- LMWH eliminated mainly by the kidneys

HELIUM

- Second lightest element to hydrogen, colourless, odourless, chemically inert and poorly soluble
- Use in airway obstruction described in 1934 by Barach (Proceedings of the Society of Experimental Biology and Medicine 1934;32: 462–464)

HENRY'S LAW

- At a particular temperature the amount of a given gas dissolved in a given liquid is directly proportional to the partial pressure of the gas in equilibrium with the liquid
- Note: as a liquid is warmed, less gas dissolves in it
- Solubility varies with the partial pressure, the temperature, the gas and the liquid

HUMIDITY

- Absolute (mg litre^{-1})

    Mass of water vapour present in a given volume of air at stated temperature and pressure
- Relative (%)

    Ratio of the mass of water vapour in a given volume of air to the mass required to saturate that given volume of air at the same temperature
- Level in upper trachea is 34 mg litre^{-1}

INFUSION FLUIDS

	0.9% Saline	4% Dextrose 0.18% Saline	Hartmann's	5% Dextrose	10% Dextrose
Glucose (g/l)		40		50	100
Na (mmol/l)	154	31	131		
K (mmol/l)			5		
Cl (mmol/l)	154	31	111		
Ca (mmol/l)			2		
Lactate (mmol/l)			29		
Calories per litre		150		188	376

Hartmann's
- Osmolarity 278 mosmol/l
- About 70% of lactate load undergoes gluconeogenesis – 2 lactate molecules $\Rightarrow$ 1 glucose
- Remainder undergoes oxidation
- Both pathways involve consumption of hydrogen ions and production of bicarbonate ions

JOULE
- Electrical units = 1 watt/second
- Mechanical units = 1 newton/metre

JOULE–KELVIN PRINCIPLE (JOULE–THOMPSON EFFECT)
- Compression of gas produces heat
- Expansion of gas leads to heat loss
- Part of reason why there must be no oil/grease in gas pipes when oxygen cylinder turned on – sudden pressurization in pipes leads to increase in temperature

KETAMINE
- Derivative of phencyclidine, highly lipid soluble
- Non-competitive antagonist at glutamate NMDA (N-methyl-D-aspartate) receptors, inhibits the facilitated state of spinal processing caused by repetitive-persistent small afferent (C fibre) input (wind up) and long-term potentiation of pain transmission
- S (+) ketamine (+ enantiomer of racemic ketamine) has 3 × the analgesic potency of the racemate

LABETALOL
- Alpha and beta-receptor blocker, 1:7 ratio

LACTATE METABOLISM
1. **Gluconeogenesis**
   $$2CH_3CHOHCO_2 + 2H \rightarrow C_6H_{12}O_6$$
2. **Oxidation**
   $$lactate + H + 3O_2 \rightarrow 3CO_2 + 3H_2O$$

- Under aerobic conditions both methods take place and in both one hydrogen ion is consumed, in turn for each molecule of hydrogen consumed one molecule of bicarbonate is formed

LAPLACE'S LAW
- Pressure gradient across the wall = tension/radius for a vessel/tube
- Pressure gradient across the wall = 2 × tension/radius for a bubble

LAW OF MASS ACTION
- The product of the concentrations of the products of a chemical reaction divided by the product of the concentrations of the reactants at equilibrium is a constant

LOCAL ANAESTHETICS
- Produce reversible block of conduction in nerves when applied directly in their vicinity
- Act by blocking sodium channels

Common chemical structure
- Aromatic ring – (ester or amide link) – amine group
- Several have a single asymmetric carbon atom and so are chiral drugs – bupivacaine, prilocaine, etidocaine

Esters – cocaine, procaine, tetracaine (amethocaine), chloroprocaine
Amides – lidocaine (lignocaine), prilocaine, bupivacaine, etc.

Amides have superseded esters because they:
- do not hydrolyse as readily, therefore being easier to heat sterilize in solution
- Have lower pKa so penetrate tissues more readily
- Are much less likely to cause allergic reactions
- LAs are weak bases with low water solubility but are formulated as hydrochloride salts which dissolve readily in water at pH 4–7. This greatly increases the ionized fraction with small amount of free base
- After injection physiological buffers raise the pH and this increases the unionized lipophylic proportion available to diffuse into the nerve. In intracellular fluid the slightly more acidic pH favours the active ionized form.

	pKa*	Relative lipid solubility	% Protein binding
Procaine	8.9	1	6
Tetracaine (amethocaine)	8.5	200	75
Lidocaine (lignocaine)	7.7	150	65
Prilocaine	7.7	50	55
Bupivacaine	8.2	1000	95
Ropivacaine	8.2	400	94

The three measures above predict the characteristics of any local agent.
* pKa = rate of onset.
Partition coefficient (lipid solubility) = absolute potency.
% protein binding = duration of action.

- However, clinically ropivacaine is said to have similar potency (not less); similar situation found with lidocaine (lignocaine) and prilocaine; possible that bupivacaine like lidocaine (lignocaine) has a vasodilator action, while ropivacaine, like prilocaine, does not, so they are held around the nerve longer
- Lower lipid solubility reduces penetration of myelin sheath and so increases differential blockade

LUNG CAPACITIES
- Volumes determined by size of the lungs and thorax

LUNG VOLUMES
- Volume changes brought about by inspiration and expiration

MALIGNANT HYPERPYREXIA
Muscle rigidity following suxamethonium
- Inability to open mouth for 2 min or easily demonstrable resistance to mouth opening for 4 min should cause concern
- 25% of those referred with jaw rigidity as a sole feature prove to be MH susceptible

Sequence of signs
- Tachypnoea
- Raised ETCO$_2$
- Progressive increase in heart rate
- Developing instability of BP and S_aO_2 falls
- Rise in body temperature
- Generalized muscle rigidity is a late sign and is accompanied by hyperkalaemia, cardiac dysrhythmias and DIC
- Speed of development is extremely variable
- Faster with volatiles (halothane worst but not much difference)

Treatment
- Stop all volatiles
- Hyperventilate on 100% oxygen
- Maintain anaesthesia with IV drugs
- Stop surgery as soon as possible
- Active cooling measures but avoid overzealous application of ice leading to vasoconstriction
- Reconstitute dantrolene and give each 20 mg bottle as it becomes available until tachycardia, etc., start to subside
- Average dose 3 mg/kg but up to 10 mg/kg has been needed
- Treat acidosis and hyperkalaemia
- Maintain diuresis

MOLE
- Quantity of a substance containing the same number of particles as there are atoms in 0.012 kg of carbon 12
- Molecular weight of substance in grams

- Contains 6.022×10^{23} molecules (Avogadro's number)
- Same as 22.4 l of ideal gas at 0°C and 1 atmosphere
  So 1 ml of halothane at 20°C gives $(1 \times 1.86)/197.4$ moles
  Or $(1.86/197.4) \times 22.4 \times 293/2731 = 227$ ml of gas at 20°C

MORPHINE
- Naturally occurring alkaloid from unripe seed pod of opium poppy
- Metabolized by glucuronidation to morphine-3-glucuronide and morphine-6-glucuronide
- M6G has analgesic and respiratory depressant effects
- M3G (predominant metabolite) is thought to be an antagonist
- Therefore analgesia related to M6G:M3G ratio

NALBUPHINE
- Potent agonist–antagonist at μ and κ receptors

NERNST EQUATION

$$EMF = (RT/ZF)\log_e(K^+in/K^+out)$$

R = gas constant, T = temperature (K), Z = valency of ion, F = Faraday constant

NERVE FIBRES

Fibre	Type	Diameter (μm)	Velocity (ms⁻¹)
Aα	Proprioception, motor	12–20	70–120
Aβ	Touch, pressure	5–12	30–70
δ	Motor to muscle spindles	3–6	15–30
Aσ	Pain, temperature, touch	2–5	12–30
B	Preganglionic autonomic	<3	3–15
C	Pain Postganglionic sympathetic	0.4–1.2	0.7–2.3

NEWTON
- Force that will give a mass of 1 kg an acceleration of $1\,ms^{-2}$ in the direction of the force
- Gravity gives an object an acceleration of $9.81\,ms^{-2}$ therefore force of gravity on 1 kg is 9.81 newtons
- Known as 1 kg weight therefore 1 newton = 1/9.81 kg.weight = 102 g weight

NITROUS OXIDE
- Dephlogisticated air – Joseph Priestly 1786
- First use by Horace Wells as an anaesthetic in 1845
- Fink described diffusion hypoxia in 1955
- Critical temperature 36.5°C
- Critical pressure 71.7 bar

- Calculate cylinder contents by weight
  1 mole N_2O occupies 22.4 l
  1 mole N_2O = 44 g
  so 44 g provides 22.4 l
  3400 g occupies $(3400/44) \times 22.4 = 17301$ at STP (i.e. at 0°C)
  at 20°C = $(1730/273) \times 293 = 1857$ ml

NYHA severity
- No functional limitation
- Slight functional limitation; fatigue, palpitations, dyspnoea or angina on ordinary physical exertion but not at rest
- Marked limitation; symptoms on less than ordinary exertion but not at rest
- Inability to perform any physical activity, with or without symptoms at rest

NONSTEROIDAL ANTI-INFLAMMATORY DRUGS (NSAIDs)
- COX_1 and COX_2 the two enzymes involved in the NSAIDs
- It is thought the balance between blockage of these determines adverse effect profile
  COX_1 found in platelets, stomach and kidney areas
  COX_2 tissue areas and is inducible, thought to produce most prostaglandins during inflammatory response
  Hence COX_1 action may bring most of the side-effects

	$COX_2 : COX_1$ ratio	$t_{1/2}$
Ketorolac	1:1	5 h
Diclofenac	1:1	2.0 h
Ibuprofen	1:1	2.4 h
Meloxicam	10:1	20 h
Celecoxib	375:1	11 h
Rofecoxib	800:1	17 h

Adverse reactions
- Renal
  Renal prostaglandins cause vasodilatation and become important with elevated levels of systemic vasoconstrictors (renin, angiotensin and noradrenaline (norepinephrine).)
  Renal blood flow becomes dependent on the vasodilatation and if removed by NSAIDs flow can be severely impaired
  Perioperative period is a particular risk especially if haemorrhage and hypovolaemia present
- Respiratory
  Bronchoconstriction can occur. Aspirin induced asthma occurs in 5–10% of asthmatics
- Gastrointestinal

Prostaglandins important in controlling production of protective mucous layer on gastric mucosa. Risks related to duration of therapy (marked increase after 5 days)
- Haemostasis
  Inhibit TXA2 production in platelets, reducing platelet aggregation
  Bleeding time increased to a variable extent – greatest with intravenous infusions

ORGAN INNERVATION
- Kidney   T10–11
- Ureter   T11–L1
- Bladder –   upper aspect   T11–L1
  trigone
  prostate   S2–S4
  urethra
- Testicle   spermatic plexus   T10
  genitofemoral   L1–2
  sacral nerves   S2–4
- Ovary and tube   T10
- Uterus   fundus   T11–L1
  cervix   S2–4
  upper vagina   S2–4

OSMOLALITY
- Moles per kg of solvent
- Measure by osmometer
- Depression of freezing point of a solution is directly proportional to its osmolality (1 mole of substance in 1 kg of water depresses the freezing point by 1.86°C)

OSMOLARITY
- Moles per litre of solution

OSTWALD SOLUBILITY COEFFICIENT
- The volume of gas which dissolves in one unit volume of the liquid at the temperature concerned

OXYGEN FLUX EQUATION
Calculate flow of oxygen to an organ
- O_2 flux = [Hb] × S_aO2 × flow + (amount in solution × flow)

PARTITION COEFFICIENT
- Ratio of the amount of substance present in one phase compared with another, the two phases being of equal volume and being in equilibrium
- Phases concerned and the temperature should be stated

PHARMACOKINETICS
- What the body does to the drug

PHARMACODYNAMICS
• What the drug does to the body

POWER
Rate of working, measured in watts
1 watt = 1 joule/second

PRESSURE
• Pressure = force/area
• Unit is pascal = 1 newton/m^2 (small so use kilopascal, kPa)
• 1 bar = 100 kPa
• 1 kPa = 10.2 cm of water
• 1 kPa = 7.5 mmHg
• Absolute pressure = gauge pressure + atmospheric pressure
• Gauge pressure = pressure above atmospheric (i.e. reads zero when at atmospheric pressure)

PROPOFOL
• 2,6-diisopropylphenol
• Alkylphenol
• Action incompletely understood but thought to work on GABA$_A$ receptor complex
• Pain on injection thought to be related to amount of propofol in aqueous phase, can be reduced by adding long chain triglycerides

PSEUDO-CRITICAL TEMPERATURE
• Applies to certain gas mixtures e.g. Entonox
• Specific critical temperature at which the gas mixture may separate out into its constituents
• −5.5°C for Entonox, most likely at pressure of 117 bar
• −30°C at pipeline pressure

RAE TUBES
• Named after inventors Drs Ring, Adair and Elwyn

RAOULT'S LAW
• The depression or lowering of vapour pressure of a solvent is proportional to the molar concentration of the solute

REYNOLDS NUMBER
• Likelihood of turbulent flow occurring can be predicted from this
• Relates velocity of flow of a gas, diameter of the tube, density of the gas and the viscosity of the gas

$$Re = (velocity \times density \times diameter\ of\ tube)/viscosity$$

ROCURONIUM
• Monoquaternary aminosteroid (similar to vecuronium but with shorter onset time)

SECOND GAS EFFECT
- Uptake of one agent may be accelerated if given in association with a high concentration of another agent
- The rapid absorption of the second gas has the effect of increasing the alveolar concentration of the first agent

SEEBECK EFFECT
- At any junction of two dissimilar metals a small voltage is produced, the size of which is dependent on the temperature
- Principle of thermocouple

SEROTONIN SYNDROME
- Results from increased synaptic levels of serotonin in the brainstem and spinal cord
- See changes in.
  — behaviour and mental state – confusion, agitation, coma
  — motor activity – rigidity, myoclonus, hyperreflexia, incoordination
  — autonomic instability – fever, diarrhoea, tachycardia, labile BP, pupillary dilatation
  — may cause high fever, seizures, nystagmus, oculogyric crises, opisthotonus, DIC, myoglobinuria, renal failure, coma and death

SLEEP APNOEA
- Cessation of airflow at the mouth and nose for at least 10 s during sleep

Obstructive
85% of cases
Absence of airflow at the mouth and nose despite respiratory movement

Central
10% of cases
Absence of airflow at the mouth and nose and no respiratory movement

Hypopnoea
Episodes of partial upper airway obstruction during sleep causing at least 50% reduction in airflow with respiratory movement resulting in a fall in S_aO_2

Mixed
5% of cases
Period of central apnoea followed by an obstructive apnoeic episode

SODA LIME
- Mixture of 90% $Ca(OH)_2$, 5% NaOH, 1% KOH plus indicator dye and silicates
- Requires presence of water for reaction
  Step 1 $2NaOH + CO_2 \rightarrow Na_2CO_3 + H_2O$
  Step 2 $Na_2CO_3 + Ca(OH)_2 \rightarrow CaCO_3 + 2NaOH$

STATISTICS
- Measures of dispersion

Range, interquartile range and standard deviation
- Measures of central tendency
  Mode, median and mean
- Confidence interval

95%	$\pm$ 2 standard deviations (actual 1.96)
99%	$\pm$ 2$\frac{1}{2}$ standard deviations (actual 2.58)

- Order statistic   rearrange sample values in ascending order of size
- Rank   position in the order statistic
- Mean $= \Sigma x/n$
- Median   middle value in the order statistic (if n is even take average of middle two)
- Mode   value with the largest frequency
- Variance

$$S^2 = \frac{\sum (x - \bar{x})^2}{n-1}$$

- Standard deviation (the square root of the variance)

$$S = \sqrt{\frac{\sum (x - \bar{x})^2}{n-1}}$$

- Standard error
  $= S/n$
- Sample range = difference between largest and smallest

STEROID COVER

Patients taking steroids

< 10 mg day	no cover required
> 10 mg day	
minor surgery	25 mg hydrocortisone at induction
moderate	usual preop steroids + 25 mg hydrocortisone at induction + 100 mg day for 24 h
major surgery	usual preop steroids + 25 mg hydrocortisone at induction + 100 mg day for 48–72 h

Patients stopped steroids

< 3 months	treat as if on steroids
> 3 months	no treatment necessary

STOICHIOMETRIC CONCENTRATION
- Concentration of any combustible vapour and oxidizing agent is the concentration at which all the combustible vapour and oxidizing agent are completed used

SUFENTANIL
- Thienyl analogue of fentanyl
- 5–10 times the potency of fentanyl because of a greater affinity for receptors

SYMPATHOMIMETICS

Receptor	Agonist	Antagonist
α_1	Methoxamine	Phenoxybenzamine
	Phenylephrine	Prazosin
α_2	Clonidine	Yohimbine
	Dexmedetomidine	

Combined antagonists are common – phentolamine, phenothiazines and butyrophenones

β_1	Dobutamine	Atenolol
β_2	Salbutamol	

Antagonists are relatively unselective

Dopaminergic receptors
- DA_1 relax renal vessels and gut smooth muscle
- DA_2 presynaptic inhibition of release of dopamine and NA
- CNS: DA_1 affect extrapyramidal activity. DA_2 affect the release of endorphins, acetylcholine, and inhibit pituitary hormone release

TACRINE
- Tetrahydroaminacrine
- Central respiratory stimulant
- Anticholinesterase effect that prolongs suxamethonium

TENSION
- The tension of a gas in solution is the partial pressure of the gas which would be in equilibrium with it

THRIFT
- Thromboembolic Risk Factors Consensus Group reported 1992
- Three groups of patients by risk factors low, moderate or high risk; those in moderate or high-risk groups need prophylaxis with heparin or warfarin

TIME CONSTANT (τ)
- Is the time at which the process would have been completed had the initial rate of change continued:

1 time constant original value falls to	37%
2 time constants value falls to	13.5%
3 time constants value falls to	5%
95% complete after 3 time constants	

TRAMADOL
- Weak opioid analgesic potency similar to pethidine
- Additional analgesic actions from inhibition of neuronal reuptake of 5 HT and noradrenaline (norepinephrine) stimulation of 5 HT release

UNIVERSAL GAS CONSTANT
- Pressure × volume/temperature (absolute) = constant
- With 1 mole of gas PV/T = R (where R is the universal gas constant)
- Therefore PV = nRT$_{(absolute)}$ (where n = number of moles)

VACUUM INSULATED EVAPORATOR

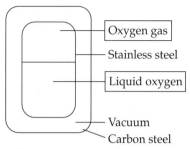

- Temperature −160°C
- Pressure 7 bar
- Oxygen flow to hospital maintains low temperature as liquid oxygen evaporates
- In periods of low demand temperature and so pressure will rise until a safety value releases some O_2 to atmosphere
- Oxygen gas (±liquid) passes through a vapourizer/heat exchanger to ensure it is raised to ambient temperature.

VALSALVA MANOEUVRE
- Forced expiration against a closed glottis

  Phase 1 increased BP (due to increased intrathoracic pressure, with temporary increased venous return)

  Phase 2 reduced BP, tachycardia (due to reduced venous return)

  Phase 3 further transient reduction in BP after expiration (due to release of intrathoracic pressure)

  Phase 4 overshoot of BP and reduced heart rate (due to increased venous return)

VAPORIZER
- Consider calculating flow through vaporizer, e.g. with halothane using fresh gas flow of 6 l/min and 1% set on vaporizer

  SVP = 32 so need 1 ml of halothane vapour to 31 ml gas to get 1%

  Flow through vaporizer will be 6000/31 = 193.5 ml/min

  Flow through bypass will be 5806.5 ml/min

  Volume of halothane will be 32% of the flow from vaporizer, i.e. 32% of 193.5 ml = 61.9 ml
- Amount of liquid halothane used

  1 ml liquid halothane at 20°C provides 22.4 × density/molecular weight × 293/273 = 227 ml therefore use 61.9/227 = 0.27 ml liquid halothane per minute

VAPOUR
- Substance below its critical temperature e.g. CO_2 critical temperature is 30.9°C so in anaesthetic practice it is a vapour, as are N_2O and cyclopropane

Index